Internal Medicine: A Comprehensive Guide to Specialized Medical Disciplines

Welcome to "Internal Medicine: A Comprehensive Guide to Specialized Medical Disciplines." This book is a comprehensive and invaluable resource that delves into the intricacies of internal medicine, offering a comprehensive exploration of the specialized medical disciplines that form its foundation. From cardiology, critical care, and endocrinology to gastroenterology, hematology, nephrology, neurology, pulmonary, rheumatology, urology, bariatrics, dermatology, epidemiology, geriatrics, hepatology, obstetrics & gynecology, osteopathy, emergency medicine, family practice, occupational & industrial medicine, physical medicine & rehabilitation, and reproductive medicine & technology, this guide provides a deep and multifaceted understanding of these critical medical fields.

Internal medicine is the foundation of healthcare, encompassing a vast array of medical disciplines that focus on diagnosing, treating, and preventing illnesses and diseases affecting adults. Each specialized medical discipline plays a vital role in the continuum of care, addressing specific health concerns and providing comprehensive solutions to enhance patient well-being.

In each chapter, this guide offers a detailed exploration of the unique intricacies of each medical specialty. We delve into the fascinating world of cardiology, where readers will gain insights into the complexities of the cardiovascular system, diagnostic techniques, and advanced cardiac interventions. The critical care chapter sheds light on the life-saving interventions provided by healthcare professionals in high-acuity settings, where timely and decisive actions are essential.

Endocrinology & metabolism takes center stage as we explore the intricate web of hormonal disorders and metabolic imbalances, emphasizing the vital role of integrated approaches in achieving optimal patient outcomes. In gastroenterology, readers will discover the diverse range of gastrointestinal disorders, diagnostic procedures, and therapeutic interventions aimed at ensuring digestive health and well-being.

Hematology unveils the fascinating world of blood disorders and hematological diseases, including advancements in hematologic oncology and blood transfusion medicine. The nephrology chapter explores the complexities of kidney function, dialysis, and renal transplantation, addressing essential aspects of kidney health and management.

The neurology chapter takes readers on a journey through the nervous system, examining the diagnostic techniques and therapeutic interventions used to address a broad spectrum of neurological disorders. Pulmonary medicine delves into the intricacies of the respiratory system, pulmonary function testing, and rehabilitation strategies to optimize lung health.

Rheumatology offers a deep understanding of rheumatic diseases and autoimmune disorders, highlighting the significance of disease management and immunosuppressive therapies. In urology, readers will explore the urinary system, urological conditions, and surgical interventions that promote urologic health.

The book further delves into bariatrics, dermatology, epidemiology, geriatrics, hepatology, obstetrics & gynecology, osteopathy, emergency medicine, family practice, occupational & industrial medicine, physical medicine & rehabilitation, and reproductive medicine & technology, offering comprehensive insights into each specialized field's unique contributions to healthcare.

Throughout the guide, evidence-based research, practical case studies, and real-world examples enrich the understanding of internal medicine's specialized medical disciplines. Aspiring healthcare professionals, seasoned practitioners, and individuals interested in the vast landscape of internal medicine will find this guide to be an indispensable resource for deepening their knowledge and appreciation of the diverse and essential medical specialties.

We invite you to embark on this journey through the comprehensive guide to specialized medical disciplines within internal medicine, gaining insights that will foster excellence in patient care, promote interprofessional collaboration, and contribute positively to the advancement of medical expertise. Together, let us delve into the intricacies of internal medicine and its specialized fields, celebrating the commitment of healthcare professionals to enhancing human health and well-being.

Introduction:

- The Significance of Internal Medicine in Healthcare

Chapter 1: Cardiology
- Understanding the Cardiovascular System and Common Disorders
- Diagnostic Techniques in Cardiology
- Cardiac Interventions and Treatment Approaches

Chapter 2: Critical Care
- Overview of Critical Care Medicine
- Management of Critical Illnesses and Trauma
- Intensive Care Unit (ICU) Interventions and

Monitoring

Chapter 3: Endocrinology & Metabolism
- Hormonal Disorders and Metabolic Imbalances
- Diagnosis and Management of Endocrine Conditions
- Integrative Approaches in Endocrinology

Chapter 4: Gastroenterology
- Digestive System Disorders and Diseases
- Diagnostic Procedures in Gastroenterology
- Therapeutic Interventions and Gastrointestinal Endoscopy

Chapter 5: Hematology
- Blood Disorders and Hematological Diseases
- Hematologic Oncology and Treatment Modalities
- Transfusion Medicine and Blood Banking

Chapter 6: Nephrology
- Kidney Function and Common Kidney Diseases
- Dialysis and Renal Replacement Therapies
- Kidney Transplantation and Long-term Management

Chapter 7: Neurology
- Disorders of the Nervous System
- Neuroimaging and Diagnostic Techniques in Neurology
- Neurological Interventions and Rehabilitation

Chapter 8: Pulmonary
- Respiratory System Disorders and Lung Diseases
- Pulmonary Function Testing and Imaging
- Pulmonary Rehabilitation and Respiratory Therapies

Chapter 9: Rheumatology
- Rheumatic Diseases and Autoimmune Disorders

- Rheumatologic Imaging and Laboratory Diagnostics
- Immunosuppressive Therapies and Disease Management

Chapter 10: Urology

- Urinary System Disorders and Urological Conditions
- Urologic Surgery and Minimally Invasive Interventions
- Management of Urinary Tract Infections and Kidney Stones

Chapter 11: Bariatrics

- Obesity and Weight Management
- Bariatric Surgery and Metabolic Interventions
- Lifestyle Modifications and Behavioral Therapy for Obesity

Chapter 12: Dermatology

- Skin Disorders and Dermatologic Conditions
- Dermatologic Procedures and Cosmetic Interventions
- Dermatopathology and Biopsies

Chapter 13: Epidemiology

- Principles of Epidemiology and Disease Surveillance
- Outbreak Investigations and Public Health Interventions
- Evidence-based Medicine and Data Analysis

Chapter 14: Geriatrics

- Aging and Age-Related Health Concerns
- Geriatric Assessment and Multidimensional Care
- Palliative Care and End-of-Life Considerations

Chapter 15: Hepatology
- Liver Function and Hepatic Diseases
- Diagnosis and Management of Liver Disorders
- Liver Transplantation and Post-transplant Care

Chapter 16: Obstetrics & Gynecology
- Maternal and Women's Health
- Obstetric and Gynecologic Surgeries
- Fertility Treatments and Reproductive Medicine

Chapter 17: Osteopathy
- Osteopathic Medicine and Holistic Approach to Patient Care
- Osteopathic Manipulative Treatment (OMT)
- Osteopathic Interventions for Musculoskeletal Disorders

Chapter 18: Emergency Medicine
- Acute Care and Emergency Interventions
- Triage and Trauma Management
- Critical Decision Making in Emergency Situations

Chapter 19: Family Practice
- Comprehensive Primary Care and Preventive Services
- Managing Chronic Diseases in Family Practice
- The Role of Family Practitioners in Healthcare Systems

Chapter 20: Occupational & Industrial Medicine
- Occupational Health and Workplace Safety
- Occupational Medicine Interventions and Injury Management
- Industrial Hygiene and Occupational Health Assessments

Chapter 21: Physical Medicine & Rehabilitation
- Rehabilitation Medicine and Functional Restoration
- Physical Therapy, Occupational Therapy, and Speech Therapy
- Assistive Devices and Mobility Aids

Chapter 22: Reproductive Medicine & Technology
- Assisted Reproductive Technologies (ART)
- In Vitro Fertilization (IVF) and Fertility Preservation
- Ethical and Legal Considerations in Reproductive Medicine

Conclusion:

- The Expansive Landscape of Internal Medicine
- The Importance of Interdisciplinary Collaboration in Healthcare
- Final Thoughts and Call to Advancing Medical Expertise

Appendix:

- Glossary of Key Terms
- List of Acronyms
- References and Recommended Readings

The Significance of Internal Medicine in Healthcare

Internal medicine plays a crucial role in healthcare as it focuses on the comprehensive and specialized care of adult patients. Internal medicine physicians, also known as internists, are highly trained medical professionals who diagnose, treat, and manage a wide range of diseases and health conditions affecting adults. The significance of internal medicine in healthcare can be understood through the following points:

1. Broad Scope: Internal medicine covers a broad range of medical conditions and diseases, including both common and complex health issues. Internists are skilled in managing chronic conditions like diabetes, hypertension, and asthma, as well as diagnosing and treating acute illnesses.

2. Primary Care Provider: Internal medicine physicians often serve as primary care providers for adult patients. They are the first point of contact for many individuals seeking medical care and play a crucial role in preventive care, health promotion, and disease screening.

3. Diagnostic Expertise: Internists are trained in comprehensive diagnostic skills, allowing them to conduct thorough evaluations and accurately diagnose complex medical conditions. Their ability to consider a patient's medical history, physical examination findings, and diagnostic test results enables timely and precise diagnoses.

4. Long-Term Patient-Physician Relationship: Internal medicine physicians often build long-term relationships with their patients, allowing for better continuity of care and a deeper understanding of the patient's medical history, preferences, and individual needs.

5. Coordinating Care: Internists coordinate care for patients with multiple health conditions or those requiring specialized medical care. They collaborate with other specialists, ensuring integrated and cohesive healthcare management.

6. Management of Chronic Conditions: Chronic diseases are a significant burden on healthcare systems. Internal medicine physicians play a vital role in managing chronic conditions effectively, promoting disease control, and preventing complications.

7. Advocates for Preventive Care: Internists emphasize the importance of preventive care and screenings to detect potential health problems early on. By encouraging healthy lifestyle changes and preventive measures, they strive to reduce the incidence of preventable diseases.

8. Adaptability to Complex Cases: Internal medicine physicians are well-versed in managing complex medical cases. Their comprehensive training equips them to handle a wide variety of conditions, making them valuable assets in both outpatient and inpatient settings.

9. Continuing Medical Education: Internists are committed to continuous learning and staying updated with medical advancements. This dedication to ongoing education ensures that they remain current with the latest evidence-based practices and treatment guidelines.

10. Critical Care Expertise: Some internists specialize in critical care medicine, providing

essential care to critically ill patients in intensive care units (ICUs). They are proficient in managing life-threatening conditions and supporting patients during their most vulnerable moments.

Overall, internal medicine plays a pivotal role in healthcare by providing adult patients with comprehensive, evidence-based, and patient-centered medical care. Internists are equipped to address a wide array of medical needs, making them essential contributors to the overall well-being of the population they serve.

Cardiology

Cardiology is a branch of medicine that focuses on the study, diagnosis, and treatment of diseases and disorders related to the cardiovascular system. The cardiovascular system includes the heart and blood vessels, and it plays a vital role in circulating blood and oxygen throughout the body. Cardiologists are medical specialists who are trained in cardiology and are experts in managing various heart-related conditions. The significance of cardiology lies in its contribution to the prevention, diagnosis, and treatment of heart diseases, which remain one of the leading causes of morbidity and mortality worldwide.

Key aspects of the significance of cardiology include:

1. Diagnosis of Heart Conditions: Cardiologists use a variety of tools and diagnostic tests to assess the health of the heart and diagnose heart-related problems. These may include electrocardiograms (ECGs or EKGs), stress tests, echocardiograms, cardiac catheterization, and more.

2. Preventive Care: Cardiologists play a critical role in promoting preventive care to reduce the risk of heart diseases. They advise patients on lifestyle changes, such as adopting a healthy diet, engaging in regular exercise, quitting smoking, and managing stress.

3. Treatment of Heart Conditions: Cardiologists are involved in the management of various heart conditions, such as coronary artery disease, heart failure, arrhythmias, valvular heart diseases, and congenital heart defects. They develop personalized treatment plans that may include medications,

lifestyle modifications, and interventional or surgical procedures.

4. Interventional Cardiology: Interventional cardiologists perform procedures like angioplasty, stent placement, and other minimally invasive techniques to treat blocked arteries and restore blood flow to the heart.

5. Electrophysiology: Electrophysiologists specialize in diagnosing and treating heart rhythm disorders (arrhythmias). They may use techniques such as cardiac ablation to correct abnormal electrical pathways in the heart.

6. Advanced Cardiac Imaging: Cardiologists use advanced imaging techniques, such as cardiac MRI and CT scans, to obtain detailed images of the heart and its structures, aiding in diagnosis and treatment planning.

7. Heart Failure Management: Cardiologists provide comprehensive care for patients with heart failure, including the prescription of medications, monitoring fluid levels, and recommending lifestyle changes.

8. Heart Health Education: Cardiologists educate patients and the general public about heart health, risk factors for heart diseases, and the importance of early detection and prompt treatment.

9. Research and Advancements: Cardiology research continues to explore new treatments, medications, and technologies to improve patient outcomes and enhance the understanding of cardiovascular diseases.

10. Collaborative Care: Cardiologists work closely with other healthcare professionals, including primary care physicians, cardiovascular surgeons, nurses, and other specialists, to ensure comprehensive and coordinated care for patients.

In summary, cardiology is a critical field in modern medicine, as heart diseases remain a significant global health concern. Cardiologists play a key role in diagnosing, treating, and preventing heart-related conditions, contributing to improved patient outcomes and overall public health. Their expertise in managing heart health is essential in reducing the burden of cardiovascular diseases and enhancing the quality of life for patients with heart conditions.

Understanding the Cardiovascular System and Common Disorders

The cardiovascular system, also known as the circulatory system, is a complex network of organs and blood vessels responsible for the circulation of blood and oxygen throughout the body. It plays a vital role in delivering oxygen and nutrients to cells, removing waste products, and regulating body temperature. The primary components of the cardiovascular system are the heart, blood vessels (arteries, veins, and capillaries), and blood.

1. Heart: The heart is a muscular organ located in the chest. It functions as a pump, continuously contracting and relaxing to propel blood through the blood vessels. It is divided into four chambers: two atria (upper chambers) and two ventricles (lower chambers). The right side of the heart receives oxygen-poor blood from the body and pumps it to the lungs for oxygenation. The left side of the heart receives oxygen-rich blood from the lungs and pumps it to the rest of the body.

2. Blood Vessels:

- Arteries: Arteries carry oxygen-rich blood away from the heart to various parts of the body.
- Veins: Veins carry oxygen-poor blood back to the heart from the body.
- Capillaries: Capillaries are tiny blood vessels that connect arteries and veins, allowing for the exchange of oxygen, nutrients, and waste products between blood and tissues.

3. Blood: Blood is a fluid connective tissue that transports essential substances throughout the body. It consists of plasma (the liquid component) and various cellular elements, including red blood cells (erythrocytes), white blood cells (leukocytes), and platelets (thrombocytes).

Common Cardiovascular Disorders:

1. Coronary Artery Disease (CAD): CAD is a condition characterized by the buildup of fatty deposits (plaque) in the coronary arteries, which supply oxygen and nutrients to the heart muscle. It can lead to reduced blood flow to the heart and cause chest pain (angina) or heart attack (myocardial infarction).
2. Hypertension (High Blood Pressure): Hypertension is a condition in which the force of blood against the walls of the arteries is consistently too high. Over time, untreated hypertension can damage blood vessels and organs, increasing the risk of heart disease, stroke, and other complications.
3. Heart Failure: Heart failure occurs when the heart is unable to pump blood efficiently, leading to a decrease in the heart's ability to supply oxygen and nutrients to the body. It can result from various heart conditions, such as CAD, heart attack, or cardiomyopathy.
4. Arrhythmias: Arrhythmias are irregular heart rhythms that can be too fast, too slow, or erratic. They can disrupt the normal electrical impulses that coordinate heartbeats and may lead to palpitations, dizziness, or fainting.
5. Valvular Heart Diseases: Valvular heart diseases involve problems with the heart valves, which regulate blood flow through the heart chambers. Conditions such as aortic stenosis or mitral regurgitation can affect valve function.
6. Peripheral Artery Disease (PAD): PAD is a condition

in which narrowed arteries reduce blood flow to the limbs, typically the legs. It can cause pain, cramping, and weakness in the legs, especially during physical activity.

7. Congenital Heart Defects: Congenital heart defects are structural abnormalities present at birth that affect the heart's structure and function. They can vary in severity and may require medical or surgical intervention.

8. Stroke: A stroke occurs when blood flow to the brain is interrupted, leading to brain damage. It can result from a blood clot or a burst blood vessel.

9. Aneurysms: An aneurysm is a weakened and bulging section of a blood vessel wall. If it ruptures, it can cause severe bleeding and life-threatening complications.

10. Deep Vein Thrombosis (DVT): DVT is the formation of a blood clot in a deep vein, commonly in the legs. If the clot dislodges and travels to the lungs, it can cause a pulmonary embolism.

These are just a few examples of common cardiovascular disorders. Proper diagnosis, treatment, and management of these conditions are essential in preserving heart health and overall well-being. Regular check-ups with healthcare professionals, including cardiologists, can help identify and address cardiovascular issues early on and reduce the risk of complications.

Diagnostic Techniques in Cardiology

Diagnostic techniques in cardiology are essential for identifying and assessing cardiovascular disorders. They help healthcare professionals gather information about a patient's heart health, function, and any abnormalities present. Some common diagnostic techniques used in cardiology include:

1. Electrocardiogram (ECG/EKG): An ECG is a non-invasive test that records the electrical activity of the heart over a period of time. It can detect abnormal heart rhythms (arrhythmias), signs of heart damage, and other cardiac issues.

2. Echocardiogram: This imaging test uses ultrasound waves to create real-time images of the heart's structure and function. It provides valuable information about the heart's chambers, valves, and blood flow.

3. Stress Test: A stress test, also known as an exercise stress test, evaluates how the heart functions during physical activity. It helps assess blood flow to the heart and can detect potential coronary artery disease.

4. Holter Monitor: A Holter monitor is a portable device worn by the patient that continuously records the heart's electrical activity for 24-48 hours. It is used to diagnose intermittent arrhythmias and other heart rhythm abnormalities.

5. Cardiac Catheterization: In this procedure, a thin tube (catheter) is inserted into a blood vessel and threaded to the heart. It allows visualization of the coronary arteries and can help diagnose blockages and other

heart conditions.

6. Coronary Angiography: This test is performed during cardiac catheterization and involves injecting a contrast dye into the coronary arteries. X-rays are then taken to visualize the blood flow and identify any blockages or narrowing.

7. Cardiac MRI (Magnetic Resonance Imaging): Cardiac MRI uses powerful magnets and radio waves to create detailed images of the heart. It provides valuable information about heart structure and function, including assessment of heart muscle viability.

8. Nuclear Stress Test: This test combines a stress test with the injection of a radioactive substance to evaluate blood flow to the heart. It is useful in diagnosing coronary artery disease and assessing heart muscle function.

9. CT Coronary Angiography: CT coronary angiography is a non-invasive imaging test that uses computed tomography (CT) to visualize the coronary arteries and detect blockages or narrowing.

10. Electrophysiological Studies (EPS): EPS is an invasive test that evaluates the heart's electrical system. It is performed to diagnose and treat arrhythmias and other electrical abnormalities.

11. Blood Tests: Various blood tests can provide valuable information about heart health, such as lipid profile, cardiac enzymes, and biomarkers related to heart damage.

12. Event Monitor: Similar to a Holter monitor, an event monitor is a portable device worn by the patient for a more extended period. It is activated by the patient when symptoms occur, allowing for the recording of heart rhythm events during specific episodes.

These diagnostic techniques, along with the expertise of

cardiologists and other healthcare professionals, play a crucial role in early detection, accurate diagnosis, and effective management of cardiovascular disorders. They help ensure appropriate treatment and care for patients with heart-related conditions, improving overall outcomes and quality of life.

Cardiac Interventions and Treatment Approaches

Cardiac interventions and treatment approaches refer to medical procedures and therapies used to manage various heart conditions and improve heart health. These interventions can be both invasive and non-invasive, depending on the specific cardiac condition and its severity. Some common cardiac interventions and treatment approaches include:

1. Medication Therapy: Medications are often prescribed to manage various heart conditions. They may include drugs to control blood pressure, reduce cholesterol levels, treat arrhythmias, and improve heart function.

2. Lifestyle Modifications: Adopting a healthy lifestyle is crucial for heart health. This includes a balanced diet, regular physical activity, smoking cessation, stress management, and maintaining a healthy weight.

3. Coronary Angioplasty: This minimally invasive procedure involves inserting a small balloon into a blocked or narrowed coronary artery and inflating it to open the artery. A stent may also be placed to keep the artery open and improve blood flow.

4. Coronary Artery Bypass Grafting (CABG): CABG is a surgical procedure used to bypass blocked or narrowed coronary arteries. It involves using blood vessels from other parts of the body to create new pathways for blood flow to the heart muscle.

5. Implantable Cardioverter-Defibrillator (ICD): An ICD is a small device implanted under the skin to monitor

heart rhythm. If life-threatening arrhythmias are detected, the ICD delivers an electrical shock to restore normal heart rhythm.

6. Cardiac Resynchronization Therapy (CRT): CRT is used to treat heart failure by implanting a special pacemaker that coordinates the contractions of the heart's ventricles, improving heart function.

7. Heart Valve Repair or Replacement: Surgical procedures are performed to repair or replace damaged heart valves, either with mechanical or biological valves.

8. Pacemaker Implantation: A pacemaker is a small device implanted under the skin to regulate the heart's rhythm and treat bradycardia (slow heart rate).

9. Heart Transplantation: In severe cases of heart failure, a heart transplant may be considered as a treatment option.

10. Electrophysiology Studies (EPS) and Ablation: EPS is an invasive procedure used to diagnose and treat abnormal heart rhythms (arrhythmias). Catheters are used to map the heart's electrical pathways, and ablation is performed to correct the abnormal rhythms.

11. Transcatheter Aortic Valve Replacement (TAVR): TAVR is a less invasive procedure to replace a diseased aortic valve using a catheter-based approach, without the need for open-heart surgery.

12. Ventricular Assist Devices (VADs): VADs are mechanical devices used to support heart function in patients with severe heart failure while awaiting heart transplantation or as destination therapy.

Cardiac interventions and treatment approaches are tailored to each individual's unique condition and medical history. They are performed by a multidisciplinary team of cardiologists, cardiac surgeons, interventional cardiologists, electrophysiologists, and other healthcare professionals. The goal is to manage heart conditions effectively, improve symptoms, enhance quality of life, and reduce the risk of complications and cardiovascular events.

Critical Care

Critical care, also known as intensive care, is a specialized area of medicine that focuses on the treatment and management of patients with life-threatening or severe medical conditions. Critical care units, commonly referred to as Intensive Care Units (ICUs), are equipped with advanced medical technology and a specialized healthcare team to provide continuous monitoring and intensive medical care to critically ill patients.

Key aspects of critical care include:

1. Patient Monitoring: Critical care patients require continuous monitoring of vital signs such as heart rate, blood pressure, respiratory rate, oxygen saturation, and temperature. Advanced monitoring devices help healthcare providers closely track changes in the patient's condition.

2. Life Support: Critical care often involves the use of life support systems, such as mechanical ventilation, to assist patients with breathing. Other life support measures include intravenous medications to support blood pressure and heart function.

3. Multidisciplinary Care Team: Critical care teams consist of various healthcare professionals, including critical care physicians, intensivists, nurses, respiratory therapists, pharmacists, nutritionists, and social workers. The team works collaboratively to provide comprehensive care and address the complex needs of critically ill patients.

4. Management of Acute Conditions: Critical care is focused on managing acute conditions such as severe

infections, organ failure, respiratory distress, cardiac emergencies, and neurological crises.

5. Medical Interventions: Critical care often involves invasive procedures, such as central line placements for administering medications and fluids, arterial lines for continuous blood pressure monitoring, and various interventions to support organ function.

6. Infection Control: Preventing and managing infections is crucial in the critical care setting, where patients are vulnerable to infections due to weakened immune systems and invasive medical procedures.

7. Nutritional Support: Critically ill patients may require specialized nutritional support to meet their increased metabolic demands and support recovery.

8. Pain Management and Sedation: Managing pain and providing appropriate sedation to critically ill patients is essential for their comfort and to facilitate medical interventions.

9. Family Support and Communication: Critical care teams also focus on providing emotional support and clear communication to patients' families, keeping them informed about the patient's condition and treatment plan.

10. Transitions of Care: As patients recover and stabilize, they may be transferred from the ICU to other specialized units or hospital wards for continued care.

Critical care is essential for patients who require close monitoring and intensive medical interventions to survive acute and life-threatening medical conditions. The specialized care provided in critical care units has significantly improved patient outcomes and survival rates for critically ill patients.

Overview of Critical Care Medicine

Critical care medicine is a medical specialty that deals with the diagnosis, treatment, and management of patients who are critically ill or have life-threatening medical conditions. It encompasses the care of patients in Intensive Care Units (ICUs) or critical care units. Critical care medicine is provided by a team of specialized healthcare professionals, including critical care physicians (also known as intensivists), critical care nurses, respiratory therapists, pharmacists, and other specialists as needed.

Key aspects of critical care medicine include:

1. Advanced Monitoring: Critical care patients require continuous monitoring of vital signs, cardiac rhythms, blood pressure, oxygen levels, and other parameters. Advanced monitoring devices and technology are used to closely track changes in the patient's condition.

2. Life Support: Critical care often involves the use of life support measures, such as mechanical ventilation to assist with breathing, hemodynamic support to maintain blood pressure, and renal replacement therapy for kidney support.

3. Multidisciplinary Team: Critical care teams are composed of various healthcare professionals who work collaboratively to provide comprehensive care to critically ill patients. This multidisciplinary approach ensures that all aspects of the patient's care are addressed.

4. Management of Complex Medical Conditions: Critical

care medicine deals with a wide range of complex medical conditions, including sepsis, acute respiratory distress syndrome (ARDS), heart failure, neurological emergencies, trauma, and post-operative care.

5. Invasive Procedures: Critical care physicians are trained in performing various invasive procedures, such as inserting central venous catheters, arterial lines, and chest tubes, as well as performing bronchoscopy and other interventions.

6. Nutritional Support: Critically ill patients often have increased nutritional requirements, and critical care teams ensure that patients receive appropriate nutritional support tailored to their needs.

7. Pain Management and Sedation: Managing pain and providing sedation to critically ill patients is important for their comfort and to facilitate medical interventions.

8. Infection Control: Preventing and managing infections is crucial in the critical care setting, where patients are at higher risk due to compromised immune systems and invasive medical procedures.

9. Communication with Families: Critical care teams provide regular updates and clear communication to the families of patients, explaining the patient's condition, treatment plan, and prognosis.

10. Transitions of Care: As patients recover, they may be transitioned from the ICU to other specialized units or hospital wards for ongoing care and rehabilitation.

Critical care medicine is a dynamic field that continuously evolves with advancements in medical knowledge and technology. It plays a vital role in improving the outcomes and survival rates of critically ill patients, making it a cornerstone of modern healthcare.

Management of Critical Illnesses and Trauma

The management of critical illnesses and trauma involves a multidisciplinary approach that focuses on providing timely and appropriate medical interventions to stabilize and support the patient. The critical care team, led by critical care physicians (intensivists), works collaboratively with various specialists to ensure the best possible outcomes for the patient. Here are some key aspects of the management of critical illnesses and trauma:

1. Rapid Assessment and Resuscitation: When a patient with a critical illness or traumatic injury arrives, the first priority is a rapid assessment of their condition. Immediate resuscitation measures are initiated to stabilize the patient's vital signs and ensure adequate oxygenation and perfusion.

2. Advanced Monitoring: Critical care patients require continuous monitoring of vital signs, cardiac rhythms, blood pressure, oxygen levels, and other parameters. Advanced monitoring devices and technology are used to closely track changes in the patient's condition.

3. Life Support Measures: Patients with critical illnesses or trauma often require life support measures. Mechanical ventilation may be necessary to assist with breathing, and hemodynamic support may be needed to maintain blood pressure and cardiac function.

4. Pain Management and Sedation: Managing pain and providing sedation to critically ill or injured patients

is essential for their comfort and to facilitate medical interventions.

5. Intravenous Fluids and Medications: Critical care patients may require intravenous fluids and medications to maintain fluid balance, correct electrolyte imbalances, and manage pain and infection.

6. Nutritional Support: Critically ill patients often have increased nutritional requirements, and nutritional support is tailored to meet their specific needs.

7. Infection Control: Preventing and managing infections is crucial in the critical care setting, where patients are at higher risk due to compromised immune systems and invasive medical procedures.

8. Surgical Interventions: Some critically ill or injured patients may require emergency surgical interventions to control bleeding, repair injuries, or remove necrotic tissue.

9. Psychosocial Support: The emotional and psychological well-being of patients and their families is an important aspect of critical care management. Providing psychosocial support helps patients and families cope with the stress and challenges of critical illness or trauma.

10. Rehabilitation and Recovery: As patients stabilize, the focus shifts to rehabilitation and recovery. Physical therapy, occupational therapy, and other rehabilitation services are provided to help patients regain function and mobility.

11. Communication with Families: Critical care teams provide regular updates and clear communication to the families of patients, explaining the patient's condition, treatment plan, and prognosis.

12. Transitions of Care: As patients recover, they may be transitioned from the intensive care unit (ICU) to other specialized units or hospital wards for

ongoing care and rehabilitation.

The management of critical illnesses and trauma requires a high level of expertise and coordination among healthcare professionals. Early recognition of the severity of the condition, timely interventions, and close monitoring are essential to improving patient outcomes. The goal is to provide comprehensive care that addresses both the immediate life-threatening issues and the long-term needs of the patient's recovery and rehabilitation.

Intensive Care Unit (ICU) Interventions and Monitoring

In the Intensive Care Unit (ICU), patients with critical illnesses or severe injuries receive specialized care and monitoring to stabilize their condition and optimize their chances of recovery. The ICU is staffed by a multidisciplinary team of healthcare professionals, including critical care physicians, nurses, respiratory therapists, pharmacists, and others, who work together to provide comprehensive care. Here are some key interventions and monitoring practices commonly employed in the ICU:

1. Mechanical Ventilation: Many ICU patients require mechanical ventilation to assist with breathing. Ventilators deliver oxygen and adjust respiratory parameters to support the patient's lung function.
2. Hemodynamic Monitoring: Continuous monitoring of blood pressure, heart rate, and cardiac output is essential for assessing the patient's circulatory status and guiding appropriate interventions.
3. Invasive Monitoring: Invasive monitoring, such as arterial lines and central venous catheters, allows for direct measurement of blood pressure, oxygen levels, and fluid status.
4. Continuous Electrocardiography (ECG): ICU patients are continuously monitored with ECG to detect any cardiac abnormalities and arrhythmias.
5. Pulse Oximetry: Pulse oximeters are used to measure the patient's oxygen saturation (SpO2) non-invasively.

6. Neurological Monitoring: Patients with neurological conditions or injuries may undergo continuous EEG monitoring or intracranial pressure monitoring.

7. Pain Management and Sedation: Pain management and sedation are carefully administered to ensure patient comfort and cooperation during medical procedures.

8. Nutritional Support: ICU patients often receive specialized nutritional support to meet their increased metabolic demands and promote healing.

9. Blood Transfusions: When necessary, blood products may be administered to stabilize the patient's hemoglobin levels.

10. Antibiotic Therapy: Broad-spectrum antibiotics may be started empirically to treat or prevent infections in critically ill patients.

11. Renal Replacement Therapy: Patients with kidney dysfunction may require continuous renal replacement therapy (CRRT) to manage electrolyte imbalances and remove waste products.

12. Wound Care: ICU patients with wounds or surgical incisions receive specialized wound care to prevent infection and promote healing.

13. Thromboprophylaxis: Measures to prevent blood clot formation (thromboprophylaxis) are implemented for patients at risk of developing deep vein thrombosis (DVT) or pulmonary embolism (PE).

14. Frequent Assessments: ICU patients are frequently assessed for changes in their condition, and interventions are adjusted accordingly.

15. Family Communication and Support: The ICU team maintains open communication with the patient's family, providing updates on the patient's status and involving them in decision-making when appropriate.

ICU interventions and monitoring are tailored to each patient's specific needs and condition. The goal is to provide timely and appropriate interventions to stabilize the patient, manage any complications, and promote recovery. Continuous monitoring allows the healthcare team to detect changes in the patient's condition promptly and initiate necessary interventions to optimize outcomes. The ICU is a high-acuity setting where patients receive specialized care, and the efforts of the healthcare team are directed toward providing the best possible care to critically ill individuals.

Endocrinology & Metabolism

Endocrinology is the medical specialty that focuses on the endocrine system, which is responsible for producing and regulating hormones in the body. Hormones are chemical messengers that play a crucial role in coordinating various physiological processes and maintaining homeostasis. Endocrinologists are medical professionals who specialize in diagnosing and treating disorders related to the endocrine system.

The endocrine system includes several glands located throughout the body, such as the pituitary gland, thyroid gland, adrenal glands, pancreas, ovaries (in females), and testes (in males). Each gland secretes specific hormones into the bloodstream, which then travel to target tissues or organs and exert their effects.

Some of the key hormones and their functions in the body include:

1. Thyroid Hormones (T3 and T4): Regulate metabolism, energy production, and body temperature.
2. Insulin: Regulates blood sugar levels by promoting the uptake of glucose into cells for energy use or storage.
3. Glucagon: Raises blood sugar levels by promoting the release of stored glucose from the liver.
4. Cortisol: Helps regulate the body's response to stress, metabolism, and immune function.
5. Growth Hormone (GH): Stimulates growth, cell reproduction, and tissue repair.
6. Estrogen and Progesterone: Regulate the menstrual

cycle and play a role in reproductive health.

7. Testosterone: Promotes the development of male sexual characteristics and supports sperm production.

Endocrinologists diagnose and treat a wide range of endocrine disorders, including:

- Diabetes Mellitus: A condition characterized by high blood sugar levels due to insulin deficiency or resistance.
- Hypothyroidism: Low thyroid hormone levels, leading to symptoms such as fatigue, weight gain, and cold intolerance.
- Hyperthyroidism: Excessive thyroid hormone production, causing symptoms like weight loss, rapid heartbeat, and heat intolerance.
- Adrenal Disorders: Including Cushing's syndrome (excessive cortisol production) and Addison's disease (insufficient cortisol and aldosterone production).
- Pituitary Disorders: Such as pituitary adenomas or hormonal imbalances.
- Gonadal Disorders: Including polycystic ovary syndrome (PCOS) and male hypogonadism.

Endocrinologists use various diagnostic tools, such as blood tests, hormone level assessments, imaging studies, and specialized stimulation or suppression tests, to evaluate hormone levels and identify endocrine disorders. Treatment may involve lifestyle modifications, hormone replacement therapy, medication, or surgical interventions, depending on the specific condition and its severity.

Metabolism, on the other hand, refers to all the chemical reactions that occur within the body to maintain life and energy balance. It includes anabolism (building up molecules) and catabolism (breaking down molecules). The metabolism of nutrients, such as carbohydrates, fats, and proteins, is essential for energy production and supporting bodily functions.

Overall, endocrinology and metabolism play critical roles in maintaining health and proper functioning of the body's systems. Endocrinologists help diagnose and manage hormone-related disorders, while metabolism impacts overall energy balance and the utilization of nutrients for growth, repair, and maintenance.

Hormonal Disorders and Metabolic Imbalances

Hormonal disorders and metabolic imbalances are conditions that arise when there are abnormalities in the production, regulation, or response to hormones in the body. These disorders can affect various systems and processes, leading to a wide range of symptoms and health issues.

Some common hormonal disorders include:

1. Diabetes Mellitus: A metabolic disorder characterized by high blood sugar levels due to insufficient insulin production or impaired insulin function (insulin resistance). There are two main types: Type 1 diabetes (an autoimmune condition where the body's immune system attacks and destroys insulin-producing cells in the pancreas) and Type 2 diabetes (insulin resistance and relative insulin deficiency).

2. Hypothyroidism: Occurs when the thyroid gland does not produce enough thyroid hormones, leading to a slowdown in metabolism. Symptoms may include fatigue, weight gain, cold intolerance, and dry skin.

3. Hyperthyroidism: The thyroid gland produces an excess of thyroid hormones, leading to an increase in metabolism. Symptoms may include weight loss, rapid heartbeat, heat intolerance, and nervousness.

4. Cushing's Syndrome: A hormonal disorder caused by prolonged exposure to high levels of cortisol (a stress hormone) in the body. It can result from the

excessive production of cortisol or prolonged use of corticosteroid medications.

5. Addison's Disease: Occurs when the adrenal glands do not produce enough cortisol and aldosterone. Symptoms may include fatigue, weakness, weight loss, and low blood pressure.

6. Polycystic Ovary Syndrome (PCOS): A common hormonal disorder in females characterized by hormonal imbalances, insulin resistance, and cysts in the ovaries. It can lead to irregular menstrual cycles, excessive hair growth, acne, and difficulty getting pregnant.

7. Growth Hormone Deficiency: A condition where the pituitary gland does not produce enough growth hormone, resulting in growth and developmental issues in children and various metabolic changes in adults.

Metabolic imbalances may involve disruptions in the metabolism of nutrients, leading to various health problems. For example:

1. Obesity: An excessive accumulation of body fat, often due to an imbalance between caloric intake and energy expenditure.

2. Hyperlipidemia: Abnormal levels of fats (lipids) in the blood, including high cholesterol and triglycerides, which can increase the risk of cardiovascular diseases.

3. Metabolic Syndrome: A cluster of risk factors that increase the risk of heart disease, stroke, and diabetes. It includes obesity, high blood pressure, high blood sugar, and abnormal cholesterol levels.

4. Malnutrition: An imbalance in nutrient intake, either insufficient or excessive, leading to nutritional deficiencies or excessive weight loss/gain.

Management of hormonal disorders and metabolic imbalances

typically involves a combination of lifestyle modifications, dietary changes, medications, and sometimes hormonal replacement therapies. For certain conditions, such as diabetes, careful monitoring of blood sugar levels and insulin administration may be required. Early diagnosis and treatment are essential to prevent complications and improve overall health and well-being. Endocrinologists and other healthcare providers play a crucial role in diagnosing and managing these disorders.

Diagnosis and Management of Endocrine Conditions

Diagnosis and management of endocrine conditions involve a comprehensive approach that includes clinical evaluation, laboratory tests, imaging studies, and individualized treatment plans. Endocrine disorders can affect various glands and hormones in the body, and the diagnostic process varies depending on the specific condition. Here are the general steps involved in the diagnosis and management of endocrine conditions:

1. Medical History and Physical Examination: The first step in diagnosing an endocrine disorder is a detailed medical history and physical examination. The healthcare provider will ask about the patient's symptoms, medical history, family history, and lifestyle factors. They will also perform a physical examination to look for signs of hormonal imbalances.

2. Laboratory Tests: Blood and urine tests are commonly used to measure hormone levels and assess how well the endocrine system is functioning. Some of the common blood tests include thyroid function tests (TSH, T4, T3), glucose tolerance tests (to diagnose diabetes), cortisol levels (for adrenal function), and hormone assays specific to the suspected endocrine disorder.

3. Imaging Studies: In some cases, imaging studies such as ultrasound, CT scans, or MRI may be used to visualize the endocrine glands and detect

abnormalities, such as tumors or cysts.

4. Dynamic Function Tests: Dynamic function tests are specialized tests used to evaluate the response of the endocrine system to certain stimuli. Examples include the ACTH stimulation test for adrenal function or the glucose tolerance test for insulin resistance.

5. Biopsy and Genetic Testing: In some cases, a biopsy may be performed to examine tissue samples from an endocrine gland. Additionally, genetic testing may be done to identify inherited endocrine disorders.

6. Specialized Consultations: Endocrine disorders often require input from different medical specialists, such as endocrinologists, gynecologists, pediatricians, and oncologists, depending on the specific condition and its manifestations.

7. Treatment and Management: Once the diagnosis is confirmed, the healthcare provider will develop an individualized treatment plan. Treatment options may include medications (e.g., hormone replacement therapy), lifestyle modifications (e.g., diet, exercise), and surgical interventions (e.g., tumor removal). The goal is to restore hormonal balance and manage the symptoms effectively.

8. Long-Term Follow-Up: Many endocrine conditions require ongoing management and monitoring. Patients may need regular follow-up appointments to assess treatment effectiveness, adjust medication dosages, and address any changes in symptoms or health status.

It is essential for patients with endocrine conditions to work closely with their healthcare team and adhere to the prescribed treatment plan. With proper diagnosis and management, many endocrine disorders can be effectively controlled, improving the patient's overall health and quality of life.

Integrative Approaches in Endocrinology

Integrative approaches in endocrinology involve combining conventional medical treatments with complementary and alternative therapies to address hormonal imbalances and optimize overall health. These approaches focus on treating the whole person, considering the interplay of physical, emotional, and environmental factors that can influence endocrine function. Here are some integrative approaches used in endocrinology:

1. Nutrition and Diet: Proper nutrition plays a crucial role in hormone regulation and overall endocrine health. Integrative practitioners may recommend personalized dietary plans that include nutrient-dense foods, antioxidants, and foods that support hormonal balance. For example, certain nutrients like zinc, magnesium, and omega-3 fatty acids can support thyroid function and insulin sensitivity.

2. Lifestyle Modifications: Stress management, regular exercise, and adequate sleep are essential components of an integrative approach to endocrinology. Chronic stress can disrupt hormonal balance, so stress reduction techniques like meditation, yoga, and mindfulness practices may be recommended.

3. Botanical Medicine: Herbal remedies have been used for centuries to support endocrine health. Some herbs have adaptogenic properties that can help the body adapt to stress and balance hormone levels. For example, ashwagandha and rhodiola are herbs often used to support the adrenal glands.

4. Mind-Body Techniques: Mind-body approaches, such as biofeedback and relaxation techniques, can help reduce stress and improve hormonal balance. These practices can positively influence the hypothalamic-pituitary-adrenal (HPA) axis, which plays a significant role in the body's stress response.

5. Acupuncture: Acupuncture is a traditional Chinese medicine technique that involves inserting thin needles into specific points on the body to stimulate energy flow. It may be used to support hormone regulation and alleviate symptoms related to hormonal imbalances.

6. Supplements: Certain supplements, such as vitamin D, probiotics, and herbal extracts, may be recommended to support endocrine function. However, the use of supplements should always be individualized and monitored by a healthcare professional.

7. Bioidentical Hormone Therapy: Bioidentical hormones are hormones that are structurally identical to those naturally produced by the body. Integrative practitioners may consider bioidentical hormone therapy to restore hormonal balance in certain cases of hormone deficiency.

8. Mindfulness-Based Stress Reduction: Mindfulness-based stress reduction programs can help individuals with conditions like diabetes and metabolic syndrome to manage stress and improve overall health outcomes.

It is important to note that integrative approaches should complement and not replace conventional medical treatments. Patients should work with a qualified healthcare professional who specializes in integrative endocrinology to develop a comprehensive treatment plan tailored to their individual needs. Integrative approaches in endocrinology can empower patients to take an active role in their health and well-being and may lead to more personalized and effective treatment outcomes.

Gastroenterology

Gastroenterology is a branch of medicine that focuses on the diagnosis, treatment, and management of disorders and diseases of the gastrointestinal (GI) tract. This includes the esophagus, stomach, small intestine, large intestine (colon), liver, gallbladder, and pancreas. Gastroenterologists are medical specialists who have extensive training in the evaluation and management of GI conditions.

Some common areas of focus in gastroenterology include:

1. Gastroesophageal Reflux Disease (GERD): GERD is a chronic condition where stomach acid flows back into the esophagus, leading to symptoms such as heartburn, regurgitation, and chest pain.
2. Peptic Ulcers: These are sores that develop on the lining of the stomach, small intestine, or esophagus. They are often caused by the bacterium Helicobacter pylori or the long-term use of nonsteroidal anti-inflammatory drugs (NSAIDs).
3. Inflammatory Bowel Disease (IBD): IBD includes conditions like Crohn's disease and ulcerative colitis, which are chronic inflammatory conditions affecting the digestive tract. Symptoms may include abdominal pain, diarrhea, and weight loss.
4. Irritable Bowel Syndrome (IBS): IBS is a functional gastrointestinal disorder characterized by abdominal pain, bloating, and changes in bowel habits without any structural abnormalities.
5. Celiac Disease: Celiac disease is an autoimmune disorder in which the ingestion of gluten triggers an

immune response that damages the small intestine lining.

6. Gallstones and Gallbladder Disease: Gallstones are hardened deposits that can form in the gallbladder, leading to pain and potential complications.

7. Liver Diseases: Gastroenterologists manage various liver conditions, including hepatitis, fatty liver disease, cirrhosis, and liver cancer.

8. Pancreatic Disorders: These include pancreatitis, pancreatic cancer, and pancreatic enzyme insufficiency.

Gastroenterologists use various diagnostic procedures to evaluate and diagnose GI conditions, such as endoscopy, colonoscopy, ultrasound, and imaging studies. They may also perform therapeutic procedures to treat certain conditions, such as removing polyps, dilating strictures, or stopping bleeding.

Treatment plans in gastroenterology often involve a combination of lifestyle changes, medications, and sometimes surgery. Dietary modifications, such as avoiding trigger foods or adopting a low-FODMAP diet, can be part of the management plan for certain conditions like IBS. Medications may be used to reduce acid production, manage inflammation, or alleviate symptoms. In more severe cases, surgical interventions may be necessary.

Overall, gastroenterology plays a crucial role in maintaining GI health and addressing a wide range of digestive disorders, helping patients achieve better gastrointestinal function and overall well-being.

Digestive System Disorders and Diseases

The digestive system is a complex network of organs that work together to break down and absorb nutrients from the food we eat. Various disorders and diseases can affect the digestive system, leading to a wide range of symptoms and complications. Here are some common digestive system disorders and diseases:

1. Gastroesophageal Reflux Disease (GERD): A chronic condition where stomach acid flows back into the esophagus, causing symptoms such as heartburn, regurgitation, and chest pain.

2. Peptic Ulcers: Sores that develop on the lining of the stomach, small intestine, or esophagus. They can be caused by Helicobacter pylori infection or the long-term use of nonsteroidal anti-inflammatory drugs (NSAIDs).

3. Inflammatory Bowel Disease (IBD): A group of chronic inflammatory conditions that affect the digestive tract, including Crohn's disease and ulcerative colitis. Symptoms may include abdominal pain, diarrhea, weight loss, and fatigue.

4. Irritable Bowel Syndrome (IBS): A functional gastrointestinal disorder characterized by abdominal pain, bloating, and changes in bowel habits without any structural abnormalities.

5. Celiac Disease: An autoimmune disorder triggered by the ingestion of gluten, leading to damage to the small intestine lining and malabsorption of nutrients.

6. Gallstones and Gallbladder Disease: Hardened deposits that form in the gallbladder, causing pain and potential complications.

7. Liver Diseases: Various conditions that affect the liver, including hepatitis (viral or non-viral), fatty liver disease, cirrhosis, and liver cancer.

8. Pancreatitis: Inflammation of the pancreas, which can be acute or chronic and may be caused by gallstones, alcohol consumption, or other factors.

9. Diverticular Disease: The formation of small pouches (diverticula) in the colon, which can become inflamed or infected, leading to diverticulitis.

10. Gastroenteritis: An infection or inflammation of the stomach and intestines, commonly known as the stomach flu, leading to symptoms like vomiting, diarrhea, and abdominal cramps.

11. Gastrointestinal Bleeding: Bleeding in the digestive tract can result from various causes, including peptic ulcers, hemorrhoids, or gastrointestinal cancers.

12. Colon Polyps and Colorectal Cancer: Polyps are growths that can develop in the colon, and some may become cancerous over time.

13. Gastrointestinal Cancers: Cancers can affect various parts of the digestive system, including the esophagus, stomach, liver, pancreas, colon, and rectum.

Treatment for digestive system disorders and diseases depends on the specific condition and its severity. It may include medications, dietary changes, lifestyle modifications, and, in some cases, surgical interventions. Early detection and timely management are essential for better outcomes and overall digestive health. Regular check-ups with a healthcare provider and seeking medical attention for persistent digestive symptoms are crucial for maintaining gastrointestinal well-being.

Diagnostic Procedures in Gastroenterology

Gastroenterologists use a variety of diagnostic procedures to assess and diagnose conditions affecting the digestive system. These procedures allow them to visualize the internal structures of the gastrointestinal tract, obtain tissue samples for analysis, and identify abnormalities or diseases. Some common diagnostic procedures in gastroenterology include:

1. Endoscopy: Endoscopy is a minimally invasive procedure that uses a flexible, lighted tube called an endoscope to examine the esophagus, stomach, and the upper part of the small intestine (upper endoscopy or esophagogastroduodenoscopy - EGD). It can also be used to examine the colon (colonoscopy). During the procedure, the gastroenterologist can take biopsies, remove polyps, and treat certain gastrointestinal conditions.

2. Colonoscopy: This procedure involves using a colonoscope to visualize the entire colon and rectum. It is commonly used for colorectal cancer screening and the evaluation of gastrointestinal symptoms such as abdominal pain, changes in bowel habits, and rectal bleeding.

3. Capsule Endoscopy: In capsule endoscopy, the patient swallows a small, disposable capsule containing a tiny camera. As the capsule travels through the digestive tract, it captures images that are transmitted to a recording device worn by the patient. This procedure is often used to examine the small intestine, which is not accessible with traditional endoscopy.

4. Endoscopic Retrograde Cholangiopancreatography (ERCP): ERCP is a procedure that combines endoscopy and fluoroscopy to diagnose and treat conditions of the bile ducts, pancreatic duct, and gallbladder. It can be used to remove gallstones, insert stents, and obtain tissue samples.

5. Endoscopic Ultrasound (EUS): EUS involves using an endoscope with an ultrasound probe at its tip to obtain high-resolution images of the digestive tract and nearby organs, such as the pancreas and liver. It helps in the diagnosis and staging of various gastrointestinal cancers.

6. Biopsy: A biopsy involves taking a small tissue sample from the gastrointestinal tract during an endoscopy or colonoscopy. The sample is then sent to a laboratory for examination under a microscope to help diagnose conditions such as cancer, inflammation, or infection.

7. Imaging Studies: Imaging techniques, such as X-rays, computed tomography (CT), magnetic resonance imaging (MRI), and ultrasound, are often used to visualize and evaluate the gastrointestinal tract and its surrounding structures.

8. Manometry: Esophageal manometry measures the pressure and coordination of the muscles in the esophagus, helping to diagnose disorders like gastroesophageal reflux disease (GERD) and achalasia.

9. Breath Tests: Breath tests are non-invasive tests used to diagnose conditions like lactose intolerance and bacterial overgrowth in the small intestine.

These diagnostic procedures help gastroenterologists accurately diagnose various gastrointestinal conditions and guide appropriate treatment plans. They are generally safe and well-tolerated, but patients should discuss the specific risks and benefits of each procedure with their healthcare providers before undergoing any diagnostic test.

Therapeutic Interventions and Gastrointestinal Endoscopy

Gastrointestinal endoscopy not only serves as a diagnostic tool but also allows for various therapeutic interventions to treat certain gastrointestinal conditions. Some common therapeutic interventions that can be performed during endoscopy include:

1. Polypectomy: During colonoscopy, polyps (abnormal growths on the inner lining of the colon) can be detected and removed using specialized instruments. Removing polyps is important for both diagnosis and prevention, as some polyps can potentially develop into cancer over time.

2. Endoscopic Mucosal Resection (EMR): EMR is a technique used to remove abnormal tissue or early-stage cancers from the digestive tract lining. It involves lifting and resecting the abnormal tissue using specialized tools.

3. Endoscopic Submucosal Dissection (ESD): ESD is a more advanced technique similar to EMR but allows for the removal of larger and more complex lesions in the gastrointestinal tract.

4. Dilation: In cases of strictures or narrowing of the esophagus, stomach, or intestines, endoscopy can be used to dilate or stretch the narrowed area using balloons or bougies.

5. Stent Placement: Stents are small tubes that can be inserted into narrowed or blocked areas of the gastrointestinal tract to maintain patency and restore

normal function. They are commonly used in the esophagus, stomach, and bile ducts.

6. Hemostasis: Endoscopy can be used to control bleeding in the gastrointestinal tract by applying various techniques, such as thermal coagulation, injection of epinephrine, or placing clips on bleeding vessels.

7. Laser Therapy: In some cases, laser therapy can be used during endoscopy to treat certain gastrointestinal conditions, such as esophageal cancer or strictures.

8. Feeding Tube Placement: Endoscopy can be used to place feeding tubes, such as gastrostomy or jejunostomy tubes, in patients who are unable to eat or swallow properly.

9. Photodynamic Therapy (PDT): PDT is a specialized treatment used to treat certain types of cancer by using a light-sensitive drug and laser light to destroy cancer cells.

10.   Argon Plasma Coagulation (APC): APC is a non-contact method used to treat certain gastrointestinal bleeding and precancerous lesions by applying ionized argon gas to the affected tissue.

These therapeutic interventions can be performed with precision and minimal invasiveness using endoscopy, allowing for quicker recovery times and reduced risks compared to traditional surgical procedures. Gastrointestinal endoscopy has revolutionized the field of gastroenterology, enabling effective treatments and improved patient outcomes for a wide range of gastrointestinal conditions.

Hematology

Hematology is the branch of medicine that deals with the study of blood and blood disorders. It includes the diagnosis, treatment, and management of conditions that affect the blood and the organs involved in its production and function. Hematologists are medical professionals who specialize in this field and are responsible for providing care to patients with various hematological conditions.

Some key aspects of hematology include:

1. Anatomy and Physiology of Blood: Hematology involves the study of the cellular components of blood, including red blood cells (erythrocytes), white blood cells (leukocytes), and platelets (thrombocytes). Understanding the normal physiology of blood is crucial in diagnosing and managing hematological disorders.

2. Hematopoiesis: Hematopoiesis is the process of blood cell formation, which primarily occurs in the bone marrow. Hematologists study the factors that regulate this process and how it can be disrupted in certain diseases.

3. Blood Disorders: Hematology encompasses a wide range of blood disorders, including anemia, leukemias, lymphomas, myelomas, bleeding disorders (hemophilia, von Willebrand disease), and clotting disorders (thrombosis, deep vein thrombosis). Diagnosis and treatment of these conditions often involve blood tests, bone marrow examinations, and specialized tests.

4. Transfusion Medicine: Hematologists play a significant role in blood transfusion services, ensuring the safe and appropriate use of blood and blood products in patients who require them due to surgeries, trauma, or certain medical conditions.

5. Hemostasis and Coagulation: The study of hemostasis involves understanding the process of blood clotting and how it can be regulated to prevent excessive bleeding or thrombosis. Hematologists are involved in managing bleeding disorders and clotting disorders.

6. Immunohematology: Immunohematology, also known as blood banking, deals with the compatibility of blood for transfusion and the identification of blood group antigens. It ensures that blood transfusions are safe and do not lead to adverse reactions.

7. Hematological Oncology: Hematological oncology focuses on the diagnosis and treatment of blood cancers, such as leukemia, lymphoma, and multiple myeloma. Hematologists work closely with oncologists to provide comprehensive care to cancer patients.

8. Bone Marrow Transplantation: Hematologists are involved in the management of patients undergoing bone marrow or stem cell transplantation, which is a treatment option for certain blood cancers and other disorders.

9. Research and Clinical Trials: Hematologists contribute to ongoing research and clinical trials to develop new therapies and improve outcomes for patients with hematological conditions.

Hematology plays a crucial role in modern healthcare, as blood disorders can have significant impacts on a patient's health and quality of life. The field continues to advance with new diagnostic tools, treatment options, and personalized therapies, making it possible to provide more effective and targeted care for patients with various hematological conditions.

Blood Disorders and Hematological Diseases

Blood disorders and hematological diseases are conditions that affect the composition, function, or production of blood and blood cells. These disorders can be broadly categorized into the following groups:

1. Anemia: Anemia is a condition characterized by a deficiency of red blood cells or hemoglobin, the protein that carries oxygen in the blood. It can result from various causes, including iron deficiency, vitamin deficiencies, chronic diseases, and genetic disorders.

2. Hemoglobinopathies: Hemoglobinopathies are inherited disorders affecting the structure or production of hemoglobin. Sickle cell disease and thalassemia are common examples of hemoglobinopathies.

3. Hemostasis Disorders: Hemostasis refers to the body's ability to control bleeding. Disorders in hemostasis can lead to bleeding disorders like hemophilia, von Willebrand disease, and platelet disorders.

4. Leukemia: Leukemia is a type of cancer that affects the bone marrow and blood. It causes an overproduction of immature white blood cells, leading to their accumulation in the blood and bone marrow.

5. Lymphoma: Lymphoma is a cancer that affects the lymphatic system, including lymph nodes and lymphoid tissues. It can be classified into Hodgkin lymphoma and non-Hodgkin lymphoma.

6. Myeloma: Multiple myeloma is a type of cancer that affects plasma cells in the bone marrow, leading to the overproduction of abnormal antibodies.

7. Myeloproliferative Neoplasms: Myeloproliferative neoplasms are a group of disorders characterized by the overproduction of blood cells in the bone marrow. Examples include polycythemia vera, essential thrombocythemia, and myelofibrosis.

8. Hemolytic Anemias: Hemolytic anemias are conditions in which red blood cells are destroyed prematurely, leading to a decreased lifespan of these cells.

9. Coagulation Disorders: Coagulation disorders involve abnormalities in the blood's ability to form clots. These conditions can lead to either excessive bleeding or thrombosis (formation of blood clots).

10. Bone Marrow Failure Syndromes: Bone marrow failure syndromes are conditions in which the bone marrow does not produce enough blood cells, leading to anemia, thrombocytopenia, and neutropenia.

11. Myelodysplastic Syndromes: Myelodysplastic syndromes are a group of disorders in which the bone marrow does not produce mature and healthy blood cells.

12. Hemophagocytic Lymphohistiocytosis (HLH): HLH is a rare and severe condition characterized by uncontrolled activation of the immune system, leading to the destruction of blood cells and organs.

Treatment for blood disorders and hematological diseases depends on the specific condition and its severity. It may include medication, blood transfusions, bone marrow transplantation, chemotherapy, radiation therapy, and other supportive measures. Early diagnosis and appropriate management are essential for improving outcomes and enhancing the quality of life for patients with these conditions.

Hematologic Oncology and Treatment Modalities

Hematologic oncology, also known as hematology-oncology, is a specialized field of medicine that focuses on the diagnosis and treatment of cancers and other disorders of the blood and blood-forming tissues. This includes diseases such as leukemia, lymphoma, myeloma, and other blood-related malignancies. Hematologic oncologists are physicians who are trained to manage and treat these conditions.

Treatment modalities for hematologic malignancies may vary depending on the specific type and stage of the cancer, as well as the patient's overall health. Some common treatment approaches include:

1. Chemotherapy: Chemotherapy is the use of powerful drugs to kill or slow the growth of cancer cells. It may be administered orally, intravenously, or through other routes.
2. Targeted Therapy: Targeted therapy involves using drugs that specifically target cancer cells or their supporting structures, minimizing damage to healthy cells.
3. Immunotherapy: Immunotherapy is a type of treatment that uses the body's immune system to recognize and attack cancer cells. It can be done through various approaches, such as immune checkpoint inhibitors and CAR T-cell therapy.
4. Stem Cell Transplantation: Stem cell transplantation,

also known as bone marrow transplantation, involves replacing damaged or cancerous bone marrow with healthy stem cells to restore normal blood cell production.

5. Radiation Therapy: Radiation therapy uses high-energy rays to kill cancer cells or stop their growth. It may be used in combination with other treatments.

6. Biological Therapy: Biological therapy involves using substances made from living organisms to enhance the body's natural defenses against cancer.

7. Hematopoietic Growth Factors: These are drugs that stimulate the production of blood cells and help patients recover from the side effects of treatments like chemotherapy.

8. Watchful Waiting: In some cases, especially for slow-growing or early-stage cancers, a doctor may recommend close monitoring without immediate treatment.

Treatment decisions are typically made through a multidisciplinary team approach, involving hematologic oncologists, radiation oncologists, pathologists, and other healthcare professionals. The goal is to tailor the treatment to the individual patient's needs and optimize outcomes while minimizing side effects.

It's essential for patients with hematologic malignancies to discuss treatment options, potential side effects, and long-term outcomes with their healthcare team. Additionally, supportive care, including pain management and psychosocial support, is an essential aspect of the comprehensive care for individuals with hematologic cancers. Regular follow-up visits and monitoring are also crucial to assess treatment response and manage any potential complications.

Transfusion Medicine and Blood Banking

Transfusion medicine and blood banking are critical areas of healthcare that focus on the collection, testing, processing, storage, and safe distribution of blood and blood products for various medical purposes. They play a vital role in supporting patient care in situations such as surgeries, trauma, cancer treatment, and managing various medical conditions. Here's an overview of transfusion medicine and blood banking:

1. Blood Collection and Donation: Blood is typically collected through voluntary blood donations from healthy individuals. Donated blood is then carefully screened for infectious diseases, blood type, and other important factors to ensure its safety and compatibility for transfusion.

2. Blood Components: After donation, whole blood is often separated into its different components, such as red blood cells, platelets, plasma, and cryoprecipitate. This allows medical professionals to provide specific components that patients may need, depending on their condition.

3. Blood Typing and Crossmatching: Before administering a blood transfusion, it is essential to determine the recipient's blood type and crossmatch it with the donor's blood to prevent adverse reactions.

4. Blood Storage and Preservation: Blood and blood components require proper storage and preservation to maintain their viability and safety. They are stored at controlled temperatures

in blood banks to ensure their effectiveness when needed.

5. Transfusion Reactions: In some cases, patients may experience adverse reactions to blood transfusions. Transfusion medicine specialists are trained to recognize and manage such reactions promptly.

6. Hemovigilance and Safety: Hemovigilance is a system that monitors and ensures the safety of blood transfusions. It involves tracking adverse events, near-miss incidents, and other transfusion-related complications to improve patient safety.

7. Blood Donation Drives: Blood banks and transfusion centers often conduct blood donation drives to ensure an adequate and safe blood supply. These efforts are particularly crucial during emergencies or times of increased demand.

8. Apheresis: Apheresis is a specialized procedure in which specific blood components are collected from a donor and the remaining components are returned to the donor. It is used to collect platelets, plasma, and other blood products for specific medical purposes.

Transfusion medicine and blood banking require strict adherence to regulatory and quality standards to ensure patient safety. The field continuously evolves, with ongoing research and advancements in blood product development, blood typing techniques, and transfusion-related technologies.

The work of transfusion medicine specialists and blood bank professionals is integral to modern healthcare, as it enables the life-saving treatment of patients who require blood transfusions and other blood products.

Nephrology

Nephrology is a medical specialty that focuses on the diagnosis and treatment of kidney-related conditions and disorders. Nephrologists are specialized physicians who are trained in managing kidney diseases, electrolyte imbalances, and disorders of fluid balance. They play a crucial role in helping patients maintain kidney health and managing chronic kidney disease (CKD), acute kidney injury (AKI), and other kidney-related issues. Here's an overview of nephrology and its key aspects:

1. Kidney Function and Physiology: Nephrologists have a deep understanding of kidney function and the role of the kidneys in maintaining the body's overall balance of fluids and electrolytes. They also study the process of urine formation and waste elimination from the body.

2. Kidney Diseases and Disorders: Nephrologists diagnose and treat a wide range of kidney-related conditions, including kidney infections, kidney stones, glomerulonephritis, polycystic kidney disease, and other congenital and acquired kidney disorders.

3. Chronic Kidney Disease (CKD): Nephrologists are experts in managing CKD, which is a progressive and often irreversible loss of kidney function. They work to slow the progression of CKD and manage associated complications.

4. Dialysis Therapy: Nephrologists are responsible for prescribing and managing dialysis therapy for patients with end-stage renal disease (ESRD) who require renal replacement therapy. Dialysis is a life-saving treatment that helps remove

waste products and excess fluids from the blood when the kidneys are no longer able to perform their function adequately.

5. Kidney Transplantation: Nephrologists are involved in the evaluation and management of patients who are candidates for kidney transplantation. They work closely with transplant surgeons to ensure successful outcomes for kidney transplant recipients.

6. Hypertension and Fluid-Electrolyte Disorders: Nephrologists are skilled in the management of hypertension (high blood pressure) and various fluid and electrolyte imbalances that can affect kidney function.

7. Research and Clinical Trials: Many nephrologists are actively involved in research to better understand kidney diseases and develop new treatment strategies. They may participate in clinical trials to test the safety and efficacy of new medications and therapies for kidney disorders.

8. Preventive Care and Patient Education: Nephrologists emphasize preventive care to protect kidney health and reduce the risk of kidney diseases. They also provide patient education on lifestyle modifications, dietary changes, and medications to manage kidney conditions effectively.

Overall, nephrology plays a critical role in maintaining kidney health, managing kidney diseases, and improving the quality of life for patients with kidney-related conditions. Nephrologists work in collaboration with other healthcare professionals, including primary care physicians, urologists, and transplant surgeons, to provide comprehensive and multidisciplinary care for patients with kidney disorders.

Kidney Function and Common Kidney Diseases

The kidneys are essential organs responsible for several vital functions in the body. Some of the key functions of the kidneys include:

1. Filtration of Blood: The primary function of the kidneys is to filter waste products, excess salts, and water from the blood to form urine. The filtered blood is then returned to the circulatory system.

2. Regulation of Fluid and Electrolyte Balance: The kidneys help maintain the balance of fluids and electrolytes in the body by adjusting the excretion of water and electrolytes in the urine.

3. Acid-Base Balance: The kidneys play a crucial role in regulating the body's pH level and maintaining a stable acid-base balance.

4. Blood Pressure Regulation: The kidneys produce renin, an enzyme that helps regulate blood pressure by controlling the volume of blood and the constriction of blood vessels.

5. Erythropoiesis: The kidneys produce erythropoietin, a hormone that stimulates the production of red blood cells in the bone marrow.

6. Vitamin D Activation: The kidneys convert inactive vitamin D to its active form, which is essential for calcium absorption and bone health.

Common kidney diseases and disorders include:

1. Chronic Kidney Disease (CKD): CKD is a progressive condition characterized by the gradual loss of kidney function over time. It can be caused by conditions such as diabetes, high blood pressure, and glomerulonephritis.

2. Acute Kidney Injury (AKI): AKI is a sudden and often reversible loss of kidney function, usually caused by severe dehydration, infections, or certain medications.

3. Kidney Stones: Kidney stones are hard mineral and salt deposits that can form in the kidneys and cause pain and blockages in the urinary tract.

4. Glomerulonephritis: Glomerulonephritis is inflammation of the glomeruli, which are tiny structures in the kidneys responsible for filtering the blood. It can be caused by infections, immune system disorders, and other factors.

5. Polycystic Kidney Disease (PKD): PKD is an inherited disorder where fluid-filled cysts develop in the kidneys, leading to kidney enlargement and potential kidney function impairment.

6. Urinary Tract Infections (UTIs): UTIs are infections that can affect the kidneys, bladder, ureters, and urethra. If left untreated, they can lead to kidney damage.

7. Nephrolithiasis: Nephrolithiasis refers to the formation of kidney stones, which can obstruct the urinary tract and cause pain and discomfort.

8. Nephrotic Syndrome: Nephrotic syndrome is a condition characterized by the leakage of large amounts of protein into the urine, leading to swelling and other complications.

9. Kidney Cancer: Renal cell carcinoma is the most common type of kidney cancer, which can originate from the cells in the lining of the kidney tubules.

Early detection and proper management of kidney diseases

are crucial to preserving kidney function and overall health. Regular check-ups with healthcare providers, maintaining a healthy lifestyle, and managing underlying conditions are essential for kidney health.

Dialysis and Renal Replacement Therapies

Dialysis and renal replacement therapies are life-saving treatments used to support individuals with kidney failure when their kidneys are no longer able to function adequately to filter waste products and excess fluids from the blood. There are two main types of dialysis: hemodialysis and peritoneal dialysis.

1. Hemodialysis: Hemodialysis is a process in which the patient's blood is filtered outside the body through a machine called a dialyzer or hemodialyzer. The patient's blood is pumped through the dialyzer, where it comes into contact with a special dialysis solution that helps remove waste products and excess fluids. After filtration, the cleaned blood is returned to the patient's body. Hemodialysis is typically performed three times a week in a specialized dialysis center or hospital.

2. Peritoneal Dialysis: Peritoneal dialysis involves using the peritoneal membrane in the abdominal cavity as a natural filter. A catheter is placed into the abdomen, and a special dialysis fluid called dialysate is infused into the peritoneal cavity. The dialysate absorbs waste products and excess fluids from the blood through the peritoneal membrane. After a period of time, the used dialysate is drained out, along with the waste products, and replaced with fresh dialysate. Peritoneal dialysis can be performed at home, giving patients more flexibility and independence.

Both hemodialysis and peritoneal dialysis have their advantages and disadvantages, and the choice of treatment depends on the patient's medical condition, lifestyle, and preferences.

3. Kidney Transplantation: For some patients with end-stage kidney disease, kidney transplantation may be a viable option. During a kidney transplant, a healthy kidney from a living or deceased donor is surgically placed into the recipient's abdomen. The transplanted kidney takes over the function of the failed kidneys, allowing the patient to regain kidney function and no longer requiring dialysis. However, finding a suitable donor and undergoing transplant surgery carry their own risks and considerations.

Dialysis and renal replacement therapies are essential for individuals with end-stage kidney disease to maintain their health and quality of life. These treatments help remove waste products, regulate fluid balance, and manage electrolyte levels in the body. It is important for patients undergoing dialysis to follow their treatment plan diligently, attend regular medical appointments, and make lifestyle modifications to support their overall well-being.

Kidney Transplantation and Long-term Management

Kidney transplantation is considered the best treatment option for many patients with end-stage kidney disease, as it offers a chance to regain kidney function and significantly improve the quality of life. However, kidney transplantation is a complex and major surgical procedure that requires careful planning, ongoing medical management, and lifestyle changes.

Kidney Transplantation Process:

1. Pre-Transplant Evaluation: Before a kidney transplant, the patient undergoes a thorough medical evaluation to assess their overall health and suitability for transplantation. This evaluation includes medical history, physical examination, blood tests, imaging, and other tests to ensure that the patient is a suitable candidate for the procedure.
2. Finding a Donor: The success of kidney transplantation depends on finding a suitable donor. Kidneys can be obtained from living donors (usually a close family member or a willing unrelated donor) or deceased donors (from individuals who have donated their organs upon their passing). Matching of blood type and tissue compatibility is critical to minimize the risk of rejection.
3. Transplant Surgery: During the transplant surgery, the diseased kidneys are removed, and the healthy donor kidney is placed into the recipient's abdomen. The new

kidney is connected to the recipient's blood vessels and ureter to allow urine to flow from the new kidney to the bladder.

Post-Transplant Care and Long-term Management:

1. Immunosuppressive Medications: After the transplant, patients are prescribed immunosuppressive medications to prevent the body's immune system from rejecting the new kidney. Compliance with these medications is crucial to ensure the long-term success of the transplant.
2. Regular Follow-up: Patients must attend regular follow-up appointments with their transplant team to monitor kidney function, manage medication dosage, and address any potential complications.
3. Lifestyle Modifications: Transplant recipients are advised to adopt a healthy lifestyle, including a balanced diet, regular exercise, and avoiding smoking and excessive alcohol consumption. These lifestyle modifications support overall health and reduce the risk of complications.
4. Infection Prevention: Due to the use of immunosuppressive medications, transplant recipients are more susceptible to infections. Taking precautions to prevent infections is essential for their well-being.
5. Monitoring for Rejection: Regular monitoring of kidney function and specific tests can help detect signs of rejection early. Prompt treatment can help prevent rejection from progressing.
6. Psychological Support: Kidney transplantation is a life-changing event, and patients may experience emotional challenges. Access to psychological support and counseling can be beneficial for coping with the transplant process and post-transplant adjustment.

7. Long-term Health Management: Transplant recipients should work closely with their healthcare team to manage other health conditions, such as diabetes or hypertension, which can impact the transplanted kidney.

It is important to note that while kidney transplantation can significantly improve the quality of life, it is not a cure for all health problems. Patients must be committed to adhering to their treatment plan and actively participate in their ongoing care to ensure the long-term success of the transplant. With appropriate care and support, many kidney transplant recipients can enjoy a better quality of life and an extended period of kidney function.

Neurology

Neurology is a branch of medicine that focuses on the study, diagnosis, and treatment of disorders and diseases related to the nervous system. The nervous system includes the brain, spinal cord, and peripheral nerves, and it plays a critical role in controlling various bodily functions and behaviors. Neurologists are medical professionals specializing in neurology and are responsible for assessing and managing conditions that affect the nervous system.

Areas of Focus in Neurology:

1. Neurological Examination: Neurologists conduct comprehensive neurological examinations to assess a patient's cognitive function, reflexes, motor skills, coordination, and sensory perception. These examinations help in the diagnosis of various neurological disorders.
2. Brain and Spinal Cord Disorders: Neurologists diagnose and treat a wide range of conditions that affect the brain and spinal cord, such as strokes, brain tumors, epilepsy, multiple sclerosis, and spinal cord injuries.
3. Peripheral Nerve Disorders: Neurologists also address issues related to peripheral nerves, which can lead to conditions like peripheral neuropathy, carpal tunnel syndrome, and sciatica.
4. Headaches and Migraines: Neurologists are often involved in the management of headaches and migraines, including diagnosing the cause and providing appropriate treatment.

5. Movement Disorders: Neurologists specialize in the assessment and management of movement disorders, such as Parkinson's disease, essential tremor, and dystonia.
6. Memory and Cognitive Disorders: Neurologists evaluate and treat patients with memory problems and cognitive disorders like Alzheimer's disease and dementia.
7. Neuromuscular Disorders: Conditions affecting the muscles and nerves, such as muscular dystrophy and myasthenia gravis, are also within the domain of neurology.

Diagnosis and Evaluation:

To diagnose neurological conditions, neurologists may use various diagnostic tools and tests, including imaging studies like MRI and CT scans, electroencephalography (EEG) for assessing brain activity, nerve conduction studies, and lumbar punctures to analyze cerebrospinal fluid.

Treatment and Management:

The treatment approach in neurology depends on the specific condition and its severity. Neurologists may prescribe medications, recommend physical therapy, provide lifestyle recommendations, and, in some cases, suggest surgical interventions to manage neurological disorders.

Collaboration with Other Specialists:

Neurologists often collaborate with other medical professionals, such as neurosurgeons, physical therapists, occupational therapists, and speech therapists, to provide comprehensive care for patients with complex neurological conditions.

Ongoing Research and Advancements:

Neurology is a rapidly evolving field, with ongoing research into the understanding of the nervous system and the development of innovative treatments. Advancements in neurology have significantly improved the quality of life for individuals with neurological disorders and continue to offer hope for further progress in the future.

Disorders of the Nervous System

Disorders of the nervous system encompass a wide range of conditions that can affect the brain, spinal cord, nerves, and other components of the nervous system. These disorders can lead to various symptoms and impact a person's ability to perform daily activities. Some common disorders of the nervous system include:

1. Stroke: A stroke occurs when there is a sudden interruption in the blood supply to the brain, leading to brain cell damage. Ischemic strokes result from blocked blood vessels, while hemorrhagic strokes occur due to ruptured blood vessels.

2. Epilepsy: Epilepsy is a neurological disorder characterized by recurrent and unprovoked seizures, which are caused by abnormal electrical activity in the brain.

3. Alzheimer's Disease: Alzheimer's disease is a progressive neurological disorder that affects memory, cognition, and behavior. It is the most common cause of dementia.

4. Parkinson's Disease: Parkinson's disease is a progressive movement disorder caused by the degeneration of dopamine-producing neurons in the brain. It leads to tremors, muscle stiffness, and difficulty with balance and coordination.

5. Multiple Sclerosis (MS): MS is an autoimmune disorder that affects the central nervous system. It causes inflammation and damage to the myelin sheath, disrupting nerve signals and leading to various

neurological symptoms.

6. Amyotrophic Lateral Sclerosis (ALS): ALS is a progressive neurodegenerative disease that affects the motor neurons, leading to muscle weakness, paralysis, and difficulty speaking and swallowing.

7. Peripheral Neuropathy: Peripheral neuropathy refers to damage to the peripheral nerves, which can lead to symptoms like tingling, numbness, weakness, and pain in the hands and feet.

8. Migraines: Migraines are severe headaches often accompanied by sensitivity to light, sound, and nausea. They may result from abnormal brain activity and changes in blood flow.

9. Traumatic Brain Injury (TBI): TBI occurs due to head trauma, leading to brain damage. The severity of symptoms can vary widely depending on the extent of the injury.

10. Spinal Cord Injury: Spinal cord injuries can result in partial or complete loss of function below the site of injury and can lead to paralysis and sensory deficits.

11. Dementia: Dementia is a broad term used to describe a decline in cognitive function, memory, and the ability to perform daily activities. It can be caused by various underlying conditions, such as Alzheimer's disease and vascular dementia.

12. Guillain-Barré Syndrome: Guillain-Barré syndrome is an autoimmune disorder that affects the peripheral nerves, leading to muscle weakness and, in severe cases, paralysis.

These are just a few examples of the many disorders that can affect the nervous system. Treatment and management of neurological disorders depend on the specific condition and may involve medications, physical therapy, occupational therapy, speech therapy, and other supportive measures. Early diagnosis and intervention are crucial in improving outcomes for individuals with neurological disorders.

Neuroimaging and Diagnostic Techniques in Neurology

Neuroimaging and diagnostic techniques play a critical role in the field of neurology by allowing healthcare professionals to visualize and assess the structure and function of the brain and nervous system. These techniques help in diagnosing various neurological disorders and monitoring their progression. Some of the commonly used neuroimaging and diagnostic techniques in neurology include:

1. Computed Tomography (CT) Scan: CT scans use X-rays to create detailed cross-sectional images of the brain and other parts of the body. They are often used to detect acute conditions such as bleeding, tumors, and skull fractures.

2. Magnetic Resonance Imaging (MRI): MRI uses powerful magnets and radio waves to generate detailed images of the brain and spinal cord. It provides high-resolution images and is useful in diagnosing various neurological conditions, including tumors, strokes, and multiple sclerosis.

3. Positron Emission Tomography (PET) Scan: PET scans involve injecting a small amount of radioactive material into the body to assess metabolic activity. They are commonly used to study brain function and to detect abnormalities in brain activity, such as in cases of epilepsy and Alzheimer's disease.

4. Single-Photon Emission Computed Tomography (SPECT) Scan: SPECT scans are similar to PET scans

but use different radioactive tracers. They are useful in evaluating cerebral blood flow and can be used to diagnose certain neurological conditions.

5. Electroencephalography (EEG): EEG measures the electrical activity of the brain through electrodes placed on the scalp. It is used to diagnose and monitor conditions such as epilepsy, sleep disorders, and brain injuries.

6. Nerve Conduction Studies (NCS) and Electromyography (EMG): NCS and EMG are tests used to assess the function of peripheral nerves and muscles. They can help diagnose conditions such as carpal tunnel syndrome and peripheral neuropathy.

7. Lumbar Puncture (Spinal Tap): A lumbar puncture involves inserting a needle into the spinal canal to collect cerebrospinal fluid for analysis. It is used to diagnose infections, inflammatory conditions, and certain neurological disorders.

8. Magnetic Resonance Angiography (MRA): MRA is a specialized MRI technique that focuses on imaging the blood vessels in the brain and neck. It is used to assess conditions such as aneurysms and vascular malformations.

9. Neuropsychological Testing: Neuropsychological tests are used to evaluate cognitive functions, memory, attention, language, and executive functions. They are valuable in diagnosing and monitoring neurological disorders that affect cognitive abilities.

10. Genetic Testing: Genetic testing can help identify genetic mutations associated with certain neurological disorders, such as Huntington's disease and muscular dystrophy.

These diagnostic techniques, combined with a thorough clinical evaluation, aid neurologists in accurately diagnosing neurological conditions and developing appropriate treatment plans for patients. Early and accurate diagnosis is crucial in improving patient outcomes and quality of life for individuals with neurological disorders.

Neurological Interventions and Rehabilitation

Neurological interventions and rehabilitation play a significant role in helping individuals with neurological disorders recover and improve their functional abilities. The specific interventions and rehabilitation techniques used depend on the type and severity of the neurological condition. Here are some common neurological interventions and rehabilitation approaches:

1. Physical Therapy (PT): Physical therapy aims to improve mobility, strength, balance, and coordination in individuals with neurological impairments. Therapists use exercises, stretches, and other techniques to address specific physical challenges.

2. Occupational Therapy (OT): Occupational therapy focuses on helping individuals regain or improve their ability to perform daily activities and tasks. Therapists work on fine motor skills, adaptive techniques, and using assistive devices when necessary.

3. Speech Therapy: Speech therapy is essential for individuals with communication disorders resulting from neurological conditions. Therapists help improve speech, language, and swallowing abilities.

4. Cognitive Rehabilitation: Cognitive rehabilitation targets cognitive functions such as memory, attention, problem-solving, and executive functions. It helps individuals with neurological deficits relearn and adapt cognitive skills.

5. Neuromuscular Electrical Stimulation (NMES): NMES involves applying electrical currents to specific muscles to improve muscle strength and function. It is commonly used in conditions like stroke rehabilitation.

6. Constraint-Induced Movement Therapy (CIMT): CIMT is used to improve motor function in individuals with hemiparesis by restraining the unaffected limb and encouraging the use of the affected limb.

7. Virtual Reality (VR) Rehabilitation: VR-based interventions are becoming increasingly popular in neurorehabilitation. They provide immersive and interactive environments to improve motor and cognitive skills.

8. Robot-Assisted Therapy: Robot-assisted devices are used to support and enhance physical therapy for neurological conditions. They provide repetitive and controlled movements to improve motor function.

9. Aquatic Therapy: Aquatic therapy takes advantage of the buoyancy and resistance of water to facilitate movement and exercises for individuals with neurological impairments.

10. Mirror Therapy: Mirror therapy is often used in stroke rehabilitation to improve motor function in the affected limb by creating the illusion of movement through a mirror reflection of the unaffected limb.

11. Biofeedback: Biofeedback techniques provide real-time feedback to individuals about their physiological responses, such as muscle activity or brainwaves, to help them gain control over these functions.

12. Medications and Pharmacological Interventions: Medications may be used to manage symptoms and slow the progression of certain neurological disorders.

Neurological interventions and rehabilitation are typically individualized to meet the specific needs and goals of each patient. The multidisciplinary approach, involving various healthcare professionals and therapists, is crucial in delivering comprehensive and effective care for individuals with neurological conditions. The ultimate goal is to enhance independence, function, and quality of life for those affected by neurological disorders.

Pulmonary

Pulmonary medicine, also known as pulmonology, is a medical specialty that focuses on the diagnosis and treatment of diseases and disorders of the respiratory system, including the lungs and airways. Pulmonologists are physicians who specialize in pulmonary medicine and provide care for patients with various respiratory conditions. Here are some key aspects of pulmonary medicine:

1. Respiratory Anatomy and Physiology: Pulmonologists have a deep understanding of the anatomy and physiology of the respiratory system, which includes the lungs, airways, diaphragm, and respiratory muscles.

2. Respiratory Conditions: Pulmonary medicine covers a wide range of respiratory conditions, including:

   - Asthma: A chronic inflammatory condition that affects the airways, causing difficulty in breathing.
   - Chronic Obstructive Pulmonary Disease (COPD): A progressive lung disease that includes chronic bronchitis and emphysema, leading to airflow limitation.
   - Pneumonia: An infection of the lung tissue, often caused by bacteria, viruses, or fungi.
   - Interstitial Lung Disease (ILD): A group of disorders that cause inflammation and scarring of the lung tissue.
   - Pulmonary Hypertension: High blood pressure in the arteries of the lungs.

- Lung Cancer: Malignant tumors that develop in the lung tissue.
- Pulmonary Embolism: A blood clot that travels to the lungs and blocks blood flow.
- Obstructive Sleep Apnea: A condition where breathing repeatedly stops and starts during sleep.

3. Diagnostic Procedures: Pulmonologists utilize various diagnostic procedures to evaluate respiratory conditions, including:
    - Pulmonary Function Tests (PFTs): Tests that measure lung function, including lung capacity and airflow.
    - Chest X-rays and CT Scans: Imaging techniques used to visualize the lungs and detect abnormalities.
    - Bronchoscopy: A procedure where a thin, flexible tube with a camera is inserted into the airways to examine the lungs and collect samples for testing.
    - Arterial Blood Gas (ABG) Analysis: A blood test that measures the oxygen and carbon dioxide levels in the blood.
    - Polysomnography: A sleep study used to diagnose sleep-related breathing disorders.

4. Treatment and Management: Pulmonologists develop treatment plans tailored to each patient's specific respiratory condition. Treatment options may include:
    - Medications: Such as bronchodilators, corticosteroids, antibiotics, and oxygen therapy.
    - Lifestyle Modifications: Including smoking cessation, weight management, and pulmonary rehabilitation.
    - Interventional Procedures: Such as bronchial stent placement, lung volume reduction

surgery, and thoracentesis.

- Mechanical Ventilation: For patients with severe respiratory failure.

5. Patient Education: Pulmonologists play a vital role in educating patients about their respiratory conditions, treatment options, and how to manage their symptoms effectively.

Pulmonary medicine is an essential branch of medicine, as respiratory conditions can significantly impact a person's overall health and quality of life. By providing comprehensive care and advanced treatments, pulmonologists strive to improve respiratory function and enhance the well-being of their patients.

Respiratory System Disorders and Lung Diseases

The respiratory system is a complex network of organs and tissues that facilitates the exchange of gases between the body and the environment. It includes the nose, pharynx, larynx, trachea, bronchi, and lungs. Various disorders and diseases can affect the respiratory system, leading to a range of symptoms and health challenges. Here are some common respiratory system disorders and lung diseases:

1. Asthma: A chronic respiratory condition characterized by inflammation and narrowing of the airways, leading to wheezing, shortness of breath, coughing, and chest tightness. Asthma symptoms can be triggered by allergens, respiratory infections, exercise, or environmental factors.

2. Chronic Obstructive Pulmonary Disease (COPD): A group of progressive lung diseases that cause airflow obstruction, making it difficult to breathe. COPD includes chronic bronchitis and emphysema. Smoking is a significant risk factor for developing COPD.

3. Pneumonia: An infection of the lungs caused by bacteria, viruses, or fungi. Pneumonia can lead to inflammation and fluid buildup in the air sacs of the lungs, causing symptoms such as cough, fever, chest pain, and difficulty breathing.

4. Bronchitis: Inflammation of the bronchial tubes, which carry air to and from the lungs. Acute bronchitis is often caused by respiratory viruses

and leads to coughing, mucus production, and chest discomfort. Chronic bronchitis is a component of COPD and involves long-term inflammation and mucus production.

5. Pulmonary Embolism: A condition where a blood clot (usually from the legs) travels to the lungs and blocks blood flow, leading to sudden chest pain, difficulty breathing, and sometimes life-threatening consequences.

6. Interstitial Lung Disease (ILD): A group of lung disorders that cause inflammation and scarring of the lung tissue. This can lead to decreased lung function and impaired gas exchange, resulting in symptoms like breathlessness and dry cough.

7. Lung Cancer: Malignant tumors that develop in the lung tissue. Lung cancer can cause a variety of symptoms, such as coughing, chest pain, weight loss, and fatigue.

8. Obstructive Sleep Apnea: A sleep disorder characterized by repeated episodes of interrupted breathing during sleep. It occurs when the muscles in the throat relax excessively, leading to airway blockage and disrupted sleep.

9. Pleural Effusion: A buildup of fluid between the layers of tissue (pleura) that line the lungs and chest cavity. It can cause chest pain, shortness of breath, and coughing.

10.   Cystic Fibrosis: A genetic disorder that affects the lungs and digestive system, causing thick and sticky mucus to build up in the airways, leading to recurrent lung infections and difficulty breathing.

11.   Idiopathic Pulmonary Fibrosis (IPF): A progressive lung disease with unknown causes that results in scarring (fibrosis) of the lung tissue, leading to breathing difficulties and reduced lung function.

12.   Tuberculosis (TB): An infectious disease

caused by Mycobacterium tuberculosis, which primarily affects the lungs but can spread to other organs. TB can cause chronic cough, fever, night sweats, and weight loss.

It is essential to seek medical attention if experiencing any respiratory symptoms or if you have concerns about your lung health. Early diagnosis and appropriate treatment are crucial for managing respiratory system disorders and lung diseases effectively. Regular check-ups and adopting a healthy lifestyle can also help prevent or manage these conditions.

Pulmonary Function Testing and Imaging

Pulmonary function testing (PFT) and imaging are essential diagnostic tools used to evaluate the function and structure of the respiratory system. They help healthcare professionals identify and monitor various respiratory conditions and lung diseases. Here's an overview of these diagnostic methods:

1. Pulmonary Function Testing (PFT): PFT measures the lung volumes and capacities, as well as the flow rates of air in and out of the lungs. It provides valuable information about how well the lungs are working and helps diagnose conditions such as asthma, COPD, restrictive lung diseases, and more. Common PFT tests include:

   - Spirometry: This test measures the amount of air you can inhale and exhale and how quickly you can do it. It helps assess airflow obstruction and lung capacity.
   - Lung Volume Measurement: This test measures the total lung capacity, residual volume, and other lung volumes to assess restrictive lung diseases.
   - Diffusion Capacity: This test evaluates how well oxygen and carbon dioxide are exchanged between the lungs and blood.

2. Imaging Studies:

   - Chest X-ray: A common imaging study used to visualize the structures of the chest and lungs. It can identify lung infections, tumors, and other abnormalities.

- Computed Tomography (CT) Scan: Provides detailed cross-sectional images of the lungs and chest, allowing for a more comprehensive evaluation of lung disorders, nodules, and masses.
- Magnetic Resonance Imaging (MRI): Utilized in specific cases to provide detailed images of lung tissues and surrounding structures.
- Positron Emission Tomography (PET) Scan: Used in certain situations to evaluate lung nodules or masses for potential malignancy.
- Ultrasound: Sometimes used for specific lung conditions, such as pleural effusion, to guide procedures or drainage.

Pulmonary function testing and imaging are complementary tools that aid in diagnosing respiratory disorders and assessing their severity. They also play a crucial role in monitoring disease progression and treatment effectiveness. The results of these tests help guide healthcare professionals in developing personalized treatment plans and providing optimal care to patients with respiratory conditions.

Pulmonary Rehabilitation and Respiratory Therapies

Pulmonary rehabilitation and respiratory therapies are essential components of comprehensive care for individuals with chronic lung diseases or respiratory conditions. These interventions aim to improve lung function, alleviate symptoms, enhance quality of life, and increase overall physical and functional capacity. Here are some key aspects of pulmonary rehabilitation and respiratory therapies:

1. Pulmonary Rehabilitation: Pulmonary rehabilitation is a multidisciplinary program that involves a team of healthcare professionals, including respiratory therapists, physical therapists, occupational therapists, and dietitians. The program is tailored to the individual's specific needs and may include the following components:

   - Exercise Training: Structured exercise programs to improve cardiovascular fitness, muscular strength, and endurance. Exercises may include walking, cycling, and strength training.
   - Breathing Techniques: Training in breathing exercises to improve respiratory muscle function, lung capacity, and control of breathlessness.
   - Education and Counseling: Information about lung disease, management of symptoms, medication use, nutrition, and

psychological support.

- Psychological Support: Addressing anxiety, depression, and stress related to living with a chronic lung condition.
- Nutritional Assessment: Evaluation of dietary habits and personalized nutritional counseling.
- Assistive Devices: Guidance on the use of assistive devices, such as inhalers and oxygen therapy.

Pulmonary rehabilitation has been shown to improve exercise capacity, reduce dyspnea (shortness of breath), and enhance overall quality of life for individuals with chronic respiratory diseases like COPD, pulmonary fibrosis, and asthma.

2. Respiratory Therapies:

- Oxygen Therapy: Supplemental oxygen is prescribed for patients with chronic hypoxemia (low oxygen levels) to improve oxygenation and reduce the workload on the heart and lungs.
- Bronchodilator Therapy: Medications that relax the airway muscles and improve airflow, commonly used in conditions like asthma and COPD.
- Inhaled Corticosteroids: Anti-inflammatory medications delivered via inhalers to reduce airway inflammation in asthma and COPD.
- Airway Clearance Techniques: Methods to help clear mucus and secretions from the airways, especially in conditions like cystic fibrosis and bronchiectasis.
- Non-Invasive Ventilation (NIV): NIV is used to support breathing in some chronic respiratory conditions, such as chronic hypoventilation or sleep apnea.

Respiratory therapies are prescribed and monitored by healthcare professionals to manage symptoms and improve lung function in various respiratory disorders.

Pulmonary rehabilitation and respiratory therapies play a crucial role in optimizing the health and well-being of individuals with chronic lung diseases. These interventions aim to empower patients to manage their conditions effectively and improve their overall quality of life.

Rheumatology

Rheumatology is a medical specialty that focuses on the diagnosis and treatment of rheumatic diseases, which are disorders that affect the joints, muscles, bones, and other connective tissues. Rheumatic diseases can be complex and often involve inflammation, autoimmune responses, and degenerative changes. Rheumatologists are specialized physicians who are trained to diagnose and manage a wide range of rheumatic conditions. Here are some key aspects of rheumatology:

1. Common Rheumatic Diseases: Rheumatologists diagnose and treat various rheumatic diseases, including:
   - Rheumatoid Arthritis (RA)
   - Osteoarthritis (OA)
   - Systemic Lupus Erythematosus (SLE)
   - Sjögren's Syndrome
   - Ankylosing Spondylitis (AS)
   - Psoriatic Arthritis
   - Juvenile Idiopathic Arthritis (JIA)
   - Gout
   - Systemic Sclerosis (Scleroderma)
   - Polymyalgia Rheumatica (PMR)
   - Giant Cell Arteritis (GCA)
   - Vasculitis (e.g., Granulomatosis with Polyangiitis, Microscopic Polyangiitis)
2. Diagnosis: Rheumatologists use a combination of patient history, physical examination, laboratory tests, and imaging studies to diagnose rheumatic diseases.

They often work closely with other healthcare professionals, such as radiologists and pathologists, to arrive at an accurate diagnosis.

3. Treatment: The management of rheumatic diseases may involve a combination of medications, physical therapy, lifestyle modifications, and patient education. Treatment goals aim to control inflammation, relieve symptoms, prevent joint damage, and improve overall quality of life.

4. Immunosuppressive Therapy: In certain rheumatic diseases with an autoimmune component, such as rheumatoid arthritis and systemic lupus erythematosus, immunosuppressive medications are prescribed to dampen the overactive immune response.

5. Biologic Therapies: Biologic agents are a newer class of medications used in the treatment of some rheumatic diseases. These medications specifically target certain components of the immune system responsible for inflammation.

6. Disease-modifying Antirheumatic Drugs (DMARDs): DMARDs are a group of drugs that slow down the progression of rheumatic diseases and help preserve joint function.

7. Joint Injections: Rheumatologists may perform joint injections with corticosteroids or other medications to relieve inflammation and pain in affected joints.

8. Multidisciplinary Approach: Rheumatologists often collaborate with other medical specialists, such as orthopedic surgeons, physical therapists, occupational therapists, and dermatologists, to provide comprehensive care to patients with complex rheumatic conditions.

9. Patient Education: Rheumatologists play a crucial role in educating patients about their condition, treatment options, and self-management strategies to improve

their quality of life.

10.   Research   and   Advancements:
Rheumatology is a rapidly evolving field, and ongoing
research continues to improve our understanding
of rheumatic diseases and develop new treatment
approaches.

Rheumatologists play a vital role in the early diagnosis
and comprehensive management of rheumatic diseases. Their
expertise helps patients effectively manage their conditions and
improve their overall health and well-being. Early intervention
and appropriate treatment can lead to better outcomes and a
better quality of life for individuals with rheumatic diseases.

Rheumatic Diseases and Autoimmune Disorders

Rheumatic diseases and autoimmune disorders are closely related, and many rheumatic diseases are considered autoimmune in nature. Autoimmune disorders occur when the body's immune system mistakenly attacks its own healthy tissues, leading to inflammation and damage. In the case of rheumatic diseases, the immune system primarily targets the joints, muscles, bones, and other connective tissues, causing various symptoms and complications.

Some common rheumatic diseases that are autoimmune in nature include:

1. Rheumatoid Arthritis (RA): RA is a chronic inflammatory disease that primarily affects the joints. The immune system attacks the synovium (lining of the joint), causing inflammation, joint pain, swelling, and eventually joint damage if left untreated.
2. Systemic Lupus Erythematosus (SLE): SLE is a systemic autoimmune disease that can affect multiple organs and tissues, including the skin, joints, kidneys, and heart. The immune system produces antibodies that target various parts of the body, leading to inflammation and organ damage.
3. Sjögren's Syndrome: This autoimmune disorder primarily affects the salivary and lacrimal glands, leading to dry eyes and dry mouth. It can also cause joint pain and inflammation in some cases.

4. Ankylosing Spondylitis (AS): AS is a type of inflammatory arthritis that mainly affects the spine and the sacroiliac joints. It results in pain and stiffness in the back and can lead to fusion of the vertebrae over time.

5. Psoriatic Arthritis: Psoriatic arthritis is a form of arthritis that affects some people with psoriasis, a skin condition. It causes joint pain, swelling, and skin symptoms.

6. Juvenile Idiopathic Arthritis (JIA): JIA is a group of autoimmune joint diseases that affect children under the age of 16. It can cause joint pain, swelling, and stiffness.

7. Systemic Sclerosis (Scleroderma): This autoimmune disease affects the skin, blood vessels, and internal organs. It leads to the hardening and tightening of the skin and connective tissues.

8. Giant Cell Arteritis (GCA): GCA is an autoimmune disease that affects medium to large arteries, particularly in the head and neck region. It can cause headaches, jaw pain, and vision problems.

9. Vasculitis: Vasculitis refers to a group of autoimmune disorders that cause inflammation of blood vessels. The inflammation can lead to damage in various organs and tissues.

It's important to note that not all rheumatic diseases are autoimmune, as some, like osteoarthritis, are primarily degenerative or mechanical in nature. However, many rheumatic diseases involve an immune system response, and understanding the role of autoimmunity is crucial for their diagnosis and treatment.

The treatment of autoimmune rheumatic diseases often involves immunosuppressive medications to reduce the abnormal immune response and control inflammation. Early diagnosis and timely intervention are essential for managing these conditions effectively and preventing complications. Rheumatologists play a key role in diagnosing and managing these autoimmune disorders and providing comprehensive care to patients with rheumatic diseases.

Rheumatologic Imaging and Laboratory Diagnostics

Rheumatologic imaging and laboratory diagnostics play a crucial role in the diagnosis and management of rheumatic diseases. These tools help rheumatologists assess the extent of inflammation, joint damage, and other changes in the body, aiding in the formulation of an accurate diagnosis and treatment plan. Here are some common imaging and laboratory tests used in rheumatology:

Imaging:

1. X-rays: X-rays are commonly used to assess joint damage in conditions like rheumatoid arthritis, osteoarthritis, and ankylosing spondylitis. They can reveal joint space narrowing, erosions, and changes in bone density.
2. Ultrasound: Musculoskeletal ultrasound is useful for evaluating joint and soft tissue abnormalities, including synovitis, tendon inflammation, and bursitis.
3. Magnetic Resonance Imaging (MRI): MRI provides detailed images of soft tissues, joints, and bones. It is often used to assess inflammation, joint damage, and complications in rheumatic diseases.
4. Computed Tomography (CT): CT scans may be used to evaluate bony changes and complications in certain rheumatic conditions.

Laboratory Diagnostics:

1. Complete Blood Count (CBC): CBC measures the number of red blood cells, white blood cells, and platelets in the blood. It can indicate inflammation and anemia, which are common in many rheumatic diseases.

2. Erythrocyte Sedimentation Rate (ESR) and C-Reactive Protein (CRP): ESR and CRP are markers of inflammation in the body. They are often elevated in conditions like rheumatoid arthritis and systemic lupus erythematosus.

3. Rheumatoid Factor (RF) and Anti-Cyclic Citrullinated Peptide (anti-CCP) Antibodies: These blood tests help in diagnosing rheumatoid arthritis and assessing disease severity.

4. Antinuclear Antibody (ANA) Test: ANA is used to screen for autoimmune diseases like systemic lupus erythematosus and Sjögren's syndrome.

5. HLA-B27 Test: HLA-B27 is associated with certain rheumatic conditions like ankylosing spondylitis and reactive arthritis.

6. Synovial Fluid Analysis: In some cases, a sample of synovial fluid from an inflamed joint may be analyzed to help diagnose conditions like gout or septic arthritis.

7. Autoantibody Testing: Various autoantibody tests are available to identify specific antibodies associated with different autoimmune rheumatic diseases.

These imaging and laboratory tests, along with a thorough physical examination and medical history, enable rheumatologists to make informed decisions about treatment options and disease management. Early and accurate diagnosis is crucial for improving patient outcomes and preventing long-term complications in rheumatic diseases.

Immunosuppressive Therapies and Disease Management

Immunosuppressive therapies are an essential component of disease management in various rheumatic and autoimmune conditions. These medications work by suppressing the immune system's activity to reduce inflammation and control the underlying disease process. They are commonly used to treat conditions like rheumatoid arthritis, systemic lupus erythematosus, psoriatic arthritis, vasculitis, and others. Here are some key points about immunosuppressive therapies and their role in disease management:

1. Mechanism of Action: Immunosuppressive drugs act by targeting different components of the immune system. They may inhibit the production or activity of immune cells and cytokines involved in the inflammatory process.

2. Types of Immunosuppressive Drugs: There are several classes of immunosuppressive medications, including corticosteroids, disease-modifying antirheumatic drugs (DMARDs), biologic agents, and targeted synthetic DMARDs. Each class has different mechanisms of action and is used for specific indications.

3. Corticosteroids: Corticosteroids like prednisone are potent anti-inflammatory drugs used to quickly control inflammation in acute flares of rheumatic diseases. However, they are not suitable for long-term use due to potential side effects.

4. Disease-Modifying Antirheumatic Drugs (DMARDs): DMARDs are a group of drugs that slow down disease progression and preserve joint function. Methotrexate, sulfasalazine, leflunomide, and hydroxychloroquine are examples of conventional DMARDs.

5. Biologic Agents: Biologic therapies target specific molecules involved in the inflammatory response. Tumor necrosis factor (TNF) inhibitors, interleukin-6 (IL-6) inhibitors, and B-cell depleting agents are some examples of biologic agents used in rheumatology.

6. Targeted Synthetic DMARDs: These newer medications selectively inhibit specific molecules implicated in the inflammatory process. Janus kinase (JAK) inhibitors are an example of targeted synthetic DMARDs.

7. Combination Therapy: In some cases, a combination of immunosuppressive medications may be prescribed to achieve better disease control and reduce the need for higher doses of individual drugs.

8. Monitoring and Safety: Regular monitoring of patients on immunosuppressive therapies is essential to assess treatment response and detect any potential side effects or complications. Patients on these medications may have an increased risk of infections and other adverse effects, so careful management is crucial.

9. Personalized Treatment: Disease management in rheumatic and autoimmune conditions often requires a personalized approach. The choice of immunosuppressive therapy depends on factors like the specific disease, disease activity, severity, and the patient's overall health status.

10. Long-Term Management: Immunosuppressive therapies are typically used for the long term in chronic rheumatic diseases. The goal is to achieve disease remission or low disease activity

while minimizing side effects.

It is essential for patients on immunosuppressive therapies to work closely with their rheumatologists and healthcare providers to optimize disease management, ensure safety, and improve their quality of life. Regular follow-up visits, medication adjustments, and lifestyle modifications are integral components of long-term disease control.

Urology

Urology is a medical specialty that focuses on the diagnosis, treatment, and management of diseases and conditions of the urinary tract and male reproductive system. Urologists are physicians who specialize in urology and are trained to provide both medical and surgical care for a wide range of urological conditions. Here are some key aspects of urology:

1. Urinary Tract: The urinary tract consists of the kidneys, ureters, bladder, and urethra. Urologists diagnose and treat conditions related to the urinary tract, such as urinary tract infections, kidney stones, urinary incontinence, and urinary obstruction.

2. Male Reproductive System: Urologists also manage disorders related to the male reproductive system, including erectile dysfunction, male infertility, prostate issues, and testicular conditions.

3. Prostate Health: Prostate health is a significant aspect of urology. Urologists screen for and treat prostate conditions, including benign prostatic hyperplasia (BPH) and prostate cancer.

4. Urologic Cancers: Urologists are involved in the management of urologic cancers, including prostate cancer, kidney cancer, bladder cancer, testicular cancer, and others. They may perform cancer surgeries and collaborate with oncologists for comprehensive cancer care.

5. Minimally Invasive Surgery: Many urological procedures can be performed using minimally invasive techniques, such as laparoscopy and robotic-

assisted surgery. These approaches offer benefits like faster recovery, shorter hospital stays, and reduced postoperative pain.

6. Stone Disease: Urologists specialize in the diagnosis and treatment of kidney stones and other urinary tract stones. They may use minimally invasive techniques to remove or break up large stones.

7. Incontinence Management: Urologists provide treatments for urinary incontinence, which is the involuntary loss of urine, often due to weak bladder muscles or other underlying conditions.

8. Pediatric Urology: Pediatric urologists focus on diagnosing and treating urological conditions in children, such as congenital abnormalities, urinary tract infections, and bedwetting.

9. Female Urology: Some urologists have expertise in female urology, addressing issues such as urinary incontinence, urinary tract infections, and pelvic floor disorders in women.

10. Preventive Health: Urologists play a role in preventive health by providing screenings, such as prostate cancer screening (prostate-specific antigen or PSA testing) for early detection and timely treatment.

Urology is a diverse and dynamic field that continues to advance with new diagnostic tools, treatment options, and surgical techniques. Early detection and timely intervention can significantly improve outcomes for many urological conditions. If you experience any urinary or reproductive health concerns, consulting a urologist is essential for proper evaluation and appropriate care.

Urinary System Disorders and Urological Conditions

The urinary system, also known as the renal system, plays a crucial role in filtering and eliminating waste products from the body. It consists of the kidneys, ureters, bladder, and urethra. Urological conditions and disorders can affect any part of the urinary system, leading to various symptoms and health issues. Here are some common urinary system disorders and urological conditions:

1. Urinary Tract Infections (UTIs): UTIs occur when bacteria enter the urinary tract, leading to infection in the bladder (cystitis), urethra (urethritis), or kidneys (pyelonephritis). Symptoms may include frequent urination, painful urination, and lower abdominal pain.

2. Kidney Stones: Kidney stones are hard mineral and salt deposits that form in the kidneys. They can cause severe pain in the back or side, blood in the urine, and difficulty urinating.

3. Bladder Infections: Also known as cystitis, bladder infections are caused by bacteria entering the bladder and can cause urinary urgency, burning during urination, and cloudy urine.

4. Benign Prostatic Hyperplasia (BPH): BPH is a non-cancerous enlargement of the prostate gland, which can lead to urinary symptoms such as frequent urination, weak urine flow, and difficulty starting urination.

5. Prostatitis: Prostatitis is inflammation of the prostate gland, leading to urinary symptoms, pelvic pain, and discomfort.

6. Urinary Incontinence: Urinary incontinence is the involuntary loss of urine, and it can be caused by various factors such as weak bladder muscles, nerve damage, or hormonal changes.

7. Overactive Bladder (OAB): OAB is a condition characterized by frequent and urgent urination, often associated with urinary incontinence.

8. Hematuria: Hematuria refers to blood in the urine, which may be visible to the naked eye (gross hematuria) or only detectable under a microscope (microscopic hematuria).

9. Interstitial Cystitis (Painful Bladder Syndrome): This chronic condition involves recurring pelvic pain, urinary urgency, and frequency.

10. Urethral Stricture: A urethral stricture is a narrowing of the urethra, leading to difficulties in passing urine and a weak urine stream.

11. Erectile Dysfunction (ED): ED is the inability to achieve or maintain an erection sufficient for sexual intercourse, and it can be related to both urological and psychological factors.

12. Testicular Conditions: Various conditions can affect the testicles, such as testicular torsion, hydrocele, varicocele, and testicular cancer.

13. Urinary Tract Obstructions: Blockages in the urinary system, such as ureteral or urethral strictures, can lead to urinary flow problems and kidney damage.

14. Bladder Cancer: Bladder cancer is the abnormal growth of cells in the bladder lining, which can cause blood in the urine and changes in urinary habits.

15. Kidney Cancer: Kidney cancer involves the

abnormal growth of cells in the kidneys and can cause flank pain and blood in the urine.

These are just a few examples of the wide range of urinary system disorders and urological conditions. If you experience any concerning urinary symptoms or have specific health concerns, it is essential to consult a healthcare professional, such as a urologist, for proper evaluation and treatment. Early detection and management can help prevent complications and improve outcomes for many urological conditions.

Urologic Surgery and Minimally Invasive Interventions

Urologic surgery involves the surgical treatment of urological conditions and disorders affecting the urinary system and male reproductive organs. Advances in medical technology have led to the development of minimally invasive techniques, which offer numerous benefits to patients, including reduced postoperative pain, shorter hospital stays, and faster recovery times. Here are some common urologic surgeries and minimally invasive interventions:

1. Transurethral Resection of the Prostate (TURP): TURP is a surgical procedure used to treat benign prostatic hyperplasia (BPH). During the procedure, a portion of the enlarged prostate is removed using a resectoscope inserted through the urethra.
2. Radical Prostatectomy: This surgery is performed to treat prostate cancer. It involves the removal of the entire prostate gland and some surrounding tissues to eliminate the cancerous cells.
3. Nephrectomy: Nephrectomy is the surgical removal of a kidney. It may be performed to treat kidney cancer, severe kidney damage, or to donate a kidney for transplantation.
4. Pyeloplasty: Pyeloplasty is a surgical procedure used to treat ureteropelvic junction (UPJ) obstruction, a condition that causes urine flow blockage between the kidney and the ureter.
5. Cystectomy: Cystectomy is the removal of the bladder

and is often performed to treat bladder cancer.

6. Transurethral Resection of Bladder Tumor (TURBT): TURBT is a procedure used to remove tumors or abnormal growths in the bladder lining.

7. Ureteroscopy: Ureteroscopy involves using a thin, flexible tube with a camera (ureteroscope) to visualize and treat conditions affecting the ureters, such as kidney stones or ureteral strictures.

8. Percutaneous Nephrolithotomy (PCNL): PCNL is a minimally invasive procedure used to remove large kidney stones by making a small incision in the back to access the kidney.

9. Extracorporeal Shock Wave Lithotripsy (ESWL): ESWL is a non-invasive procedure that uses shock waves to break down kidney stones into smaller pieces that can be easily passed in the urine.

10. Laparoscopic Urologic Surgery: Laparoscopic techniques involve making small incisions and using specialized instruments and a camera to perform urological surgeries, such as nephrectomy or partial nephrectomy.

11. Robotic-Assisted Urologic Surgery: Robotic-assisted surgery combines laparoscopic techniques with robotic technology to enhance precision and control during urologic procedures.

12. Prostate Seed Implantation (Brachytherapy): Brachytherapy is a type of radiation therapy used to treat prostate cancer by placing tiny radioactive seeds directly into the prostate gland.

13. Urethral Sling Surgery: This surgical procedure is used to treat stress urinary incontinence in women by supporting the urethra and bladder neck.

Minimally invasive interventions in urology have revolutionized the field, providing patients with effective treatment options and faster recovery times. However, not all urologic conditions can be treated with minimally invasive techniques, and some cases may still require traditional open surgeries. A urologist will assess each patient's condition and recommend the most appropriate treatment approach based on individual needs and medical factors.

Management of Urinary Tract Infections and Kidney Stones

Management of Urinary Tract Infections (UTIs):

1. Antibiotic Therapy: UTIs are commonly treated with antibiotics. The choice of antibiotic depends on the type of bacteria causing the infection and its sensitivity to specific drugs. Commonly prescribed antibiotics include trimethoprim-sulfamethoxazole, nitrofurantoin, ciprofloxacin, and amoxicillin.

2. Fluid Intake: Drinking plenty of water helps flush out bacteria from the urinary tract and promotes healing. Increased fluid intake is especially important during a UTI.

3. Pain Relief: Over-the-counter pain relievers like acetaminophen or ibuprofen can help alleviate pain and discomfort associated with UTIs.

4. Urinary Alkalinizers: Some patients may benefit from urinary alkalinizers, which make the urine less acidic and may help ease symptoms.

5. Prevention: To prevent UTIs, individuals should practice good hygiene, empty their bladder regularly, avoid holding in urine for extended periods, and wipe from front to back after using the bathroom.

Management of Kidney Stones:

1. Pain Management: Pain caused by kidney stones is often intense and requires immediate relief. Over-the-counter pain medications like ibuprofen or

prescription pain medications can help manage pain.

2. Hydration: Drinking ample fluids is essential to flush out small kidney stones and prevent further stone formation. Water is the best choice, but citrus juices may also be beneficial.

3. Medications: Depending on the type and cause of kidney stones, medications may be prescribed to help dissolve or prevent stone formation. For example, alpha-blockers can help relax the muscles in the urinary tract, allowing stones to pass more easily.

4. Lithotripsy: Extracorporeal Shock Wave Lithotripsy (ESWL) is a non-invasive procedure that uses shock waves to break kidney stones into smaller pieces, making them easier to pass.

5. Ureteroscopy and Laser Lithotripsy: Ureteroscopy is a procedure where a thin scope is inserted through the urethra and bladder to directly visualize and remove or break up stones in the ureters or kidneys using laser energy.

6. Percutaneous Nephrolithotomy (PCNL): PCNL is a minimally invasive procedure in which a small incision is made in the back to access and remove larger kidney stones.

7. Prevention: Lifestyle changes and dietary modifications may be recommended to prevent the recurrence of kidney stones. These may include reducing sodium intake, avoiding excessive animal protein, maintaining a balanced diet, and staying well-hydrated.

Both UTIs and kidney stones can cause significant discomfort and complications if left untreated. It is crucial to seek medical attention promptly for appropriate diagnosis and management. The management approach may vary based on the severity and complexity of the condition, so consulting with a healthcare professional is essential for personalized care.

Bariatrics

Bariatrics is the branch of medicine that deals with the management and treatment of obesity and related health conditions. It involves the study of the causes of obesity, the impact of obesity on health, and the development of strategies for weight management and weight loss. Bariatric medicine is a specialized field that focuses on providing comprehensive care for individuals struggling with obesity.

Obesity is a complex medical condition characterized by an excess accumulation of body fat that can have significant adverse effects on overall health. It is associated with an increased risk of various chronic diseases, including type 2 diabetes, heart disease, hypertension, sleep apnea, certain cancers, and joint problems, among others.

The management of obesity typically involves a multidisciplinary approach, including the collaboration of healthcare professionals such as:

1. Bariatric Physicians: Medical doctors specialized in bariatric medicine who diagnose and treat obesity and related health conditions. They create personalized weight management plans and may prescribe medications for weight loss.
2. Dietitians/Nutritionists: These professionals provide dietary counseling and create nutrition plans tailored to an individual's needs and weight loss goals.
3. Exercise Physiologists/Physical Therapists: They design safe and effective exercise programs to help individuals increase physical activity and improve

overall fitness.

4. Behavioral Therapists/Counselors: These professionals work with individuals to address emotional and psychological factors contributing to overeating or unhealthy eating habits.

5. Bariatric Surgeons: In severe cases of obesity, bariatric surgery may be considered as a treatment option. Bariatric surgeons specialize in performing weight loss surgeries, such as gastric bypass, gastric sleeve, and adjustable gastric banding.

Bariatric interventions aim to help individuals achieve and maintain a healthier weight, reduce obesity-related health risks, and improve overall quality of life. Treatment plans may include dietary changes, physical activity, behavior modification, and, in some cases, medical or surgical interventions.

It is important to note that successful long-term weight management often requires ongoing support and lifestyle changes. Bariatric medicine focuses on providing comprehensive care and support to help individuals achieve sustainable weight loss and improve their overall health.

Obesity and Weight Management

Obesity is a complex medical condition characterized by excessive body fat accumulation that can have significant health implications. It is commonly measured using the body mass index (BMI), which is calculated by dividing a person's weight in kilograms by the square of their height in meters (BMI = weight in kg / (height in meters)^2). A BMI of 30 or higher is generally considered indicative of obesity.

Causes of Obesity: Obesity is caused by a combination of genetic, environmental, and lifestyle factors. Some of the main contributors to obesity include:

1. Poor Diet: Consuming high-calorie, processed, and unhealthy foods can lead to weight gain.
2. Lack of Physical Activity: Sedentary lifestyles and insufficient physical activity can contribute to obesity.
3. Genetics: Certain genes may predispose individuals to obesity, making it easier for them to gain weight.
4. Hormonal Imbalances: Hormonal disorders or imbalances can affect metabolism and lead to weight gain.
5. Psychological Factors: Emotional eating, stress, and other psychological factors can influence eating habits and contribute to obesity.

Health Risks of Obesity: Obesity is associated with a range of health risks and medical conditions, including:

1. Type 2 Diabetes: Obesity is a significant risk factor for developing insulin resistance and type 2 diabetes.

2. Cardiovascular Diseases: Obesity can increase the risk of heart disease, high blood pressure, and stroke.
3. Sleep Apnea: Excess body fat can lead to breathing difficulties during sleep, resulting in sleep apnea.
4. Joint Problems: Obesity puts extra strain on the joints, leading to conditions such as osteoarthritis.
5. Respiratory Problems: Obesity can affect lung function and increase the risk of respiratory disorders.
6. Certain Cancers: Obese individuals have a higher risk of developing certain types of cancer, including breast, colon, and kidney cancer.

Weight Management Strategies: Effective weight management involves a combination of healthy eating, physical activity, and lifestyle changes. Some strategies to manage weight include:

1. Balanced Diet: Adopting a balanced and nutritious diet with appropriate portion sizes is crucial for weight management.
2. Regular Exercise: Engaging in regular physical activity can help burn calories and support weight loss.
3. Behavior Modification: Identifying and addressing emotional eating patterns and triggers can aid in sustainable weight management.
4. Support Groups: Joining support groups or seeking professional counseling can provide guidance and encouragement in the weight loss journey.
5. Medical Interventions: In some cases, healthcare providers may recommend medications or weight loss surgery for individuals with severe obesity.

It is essential to approach weight management as a long-term commitment to a healthier lifestyle. Sustainable weight loss is often gradual and requires patience and dedication. Seeking guidance from healthcare professionals, such as dietitians, nutritionists, or bariatric specialists, can provide personalized and evidence-based strategies for successful weight management and improved overall health.

Bariatric Surgery and Metabolic Interventions

Bariatric surgery is a type of weight loss surgery that involves making changes to the digestive system to help individuals with severe obesity lose weight and improve their health. These surgeries work by limiting the amount of food the stomach can hold or by reducing the absorption of nutrients in the small intestine. Bariatric surgery is considered when other weight loss methods, such as diet and exercise, have not been successful or when obesity-related health conditions are severe.

There are several types of bariatric surgeries, including:

1. Gastric Bypass: This surgery involves creating a small pouch at the top of the stomach and connecting it directly to the small intestine. This limits the amount of food the stomach can hold and reduces nutrient absorption.
2. Sleeve Gastrectomy: In this procedure, a large portion of the stomach is removed, leaving a small, banana-shaped sleeve. This restricts the amount of food the stomach can hold.
3. Adjustable Gastric Banding: A band is placed around the upper part of the stomach, creating a small pouch. The band can be adjusted to control the size of the opening between the pouch and the rest of the stomach.
4. Biliopancreatic Diversion with Duodenal Switch (BPD/DS): This surgery involves a combination of restrictive

and malabsorptive procedures, limiting both food intake and nutrient absorption.

Bariatric surgery is not a cosmetic procedure and should only be considered for individuals with a BMI over 40 or a BMI over 35 with significant obesity-related health conditions, such as type 2 diabetes, high blood pressure, or sleep apnea.

Metabolic interventions, on the other hand, refer to non-surgical approaches aimed at addressing the metabolic imbalances associated with obesity and related health conditions. These interventions may include lifestyle changes, dietary modifications, physical activity, behavior therapy, and medical treatments to manage obesity and its health consequences.

Bariatric surgery and metabolic interventions are considered effective in promoting significant and sustained weight loss, improving metabolic health, and reducing the risk of obesity-related diseases. However, they are not without risks and potential complications, and they should be undertaken with careful consideration and under the guidance of experienced healthcare professionals.

Before considering bariatric surgery or metabolic interventions, individuals should undergo a thorough evaluation by a qualified healthcare team to assess their overall health, understand the risks and benefits, and establish realistic expectations for the outcomes. Additionally, long-term follow-up and support are essential to ensure successful weight management and overall health improvement after these interventions.

Lifestyle Modifications and Behavioral Therapy for Obesity

Lifestyle modifications and behavioral therapy are crucial components of obesity management. They focus on helping individuals make sustainable changes to their eating habits, physical activity levels, and overall behavior to achieve and maintain a healthy weight. These approaches are often recommended as the first-line treatment for obesity, either alone or in combination with other interventions like medical treatments or bariatric surgery. Here are some key elements of lifestyle modifications and behavioral therapy for obesity:

1. Dietary Changes: A balanced and nutritious diet is essential for weight management. The focus is on consuming a variety of nutrient-dense foods, including fruits, vegetables, whole grains, lean proteins, and healthy fats. Portion control and mindful eating are also emphasized.

2. Physical Activity: Regular physical activity is vital for burning calories and maintaining a healthy weight. Incorporating aerobic exercises, strength training, and flexibility exercises into the daily routine can help increase energy expenditure.

3. Behavior Modification: Identifying and changing unhealthy behaviors that contribute to overeating or sedentary habits is a key aspect of behavioral therapy. Techniques like self-monitoring, goal setting, and problem-solving are used to address emotional eating, food cravings, and other behavioral challenges.

4. Setting Realistic Goals: Encouraging individuals to set achievable, realistic, and measurable goals is important for sustained progress. Celebrating small successes can help build motivation and confidence.

5. Stress Management: Stress and emotional factors can contribute to overeating or unhealthy eating patterns. Stress-reduction techniques such as meditation, yoga, or relaxation exercises can be helpful.

6. Social Support: Engaging in weight loss programs that offer group support or involving family and friends in the process can provide valuable encouragement and motivation.

7. Sleep and Rest: Adequate sleep and rest are essential for overall health and can positively influence eating behaviors and metabolism.

8. Long-Term Approach: Lifestyle modifications and behavioral therapy should be viewed as a long-term commitment to health. Consistency and patience are necessary as sustainable changes take time to yield results.

9. Professional Support: Working with a healthcare professional, such as a registered dietitian, nutritionist, or behavior therapist, can provide personalized guidance and support throughout the weight loss journey.

It's important to note that each individual's needs and circumstances are unique, and what works for one person may not work for another. Customized and patient-centered approaches are crucial for successful weight management and improving overall health. If individuals face challenges in achieving their weight loss goals or have underlying medical conditions, they should consult a healthcare provider to develop an appropriate and effective plan.

Dermatology

Dermatology is the branch of medicine that focuses on the diagnosis and treatment of conditions related to the skin, hair, nails, and mucous membranes. Dermatologists are medical professionals specialized in this field and deal with a wide range of skin-related issues. Here are some key aspects of dermatology:

1. Skin Conditions: Dermatologists diagnose and treat various skin conditions, including acne, eczema, psoriasis, rosacea, dermatitis, hives, and fungal infections.
2. Skin Cancer: They play a crucial role in identifying and treating skin cancers, such as melanoma, basal cell carcinoma, and squamous cell carcinoma. Regular skin screenings are essential for early detection and treatment.
3. Cosmetic Dermatology: Some dermatologists also provide cosmetic procedures to enhance the appearance of the skin, including Botox injections, dermal fillers, chemical peels, laser treatments, and microdermabrasion.
4. Allergies and Sensitivities: Dermatologists diagnose and manage allergic reactions, contact dermatitis, and other skin sensitivities triggered by certain substances.
5. Hair and Nail Disorders: They also address issues related to hair loss (alopecia) and nail problems like infections, discoloration, and ingrown nails.
6. Chronic Skin Conditions: Dermatologists assist patients in managing chronic skin conditions that

require ongoing care and treatment.

7. Pediatric Dermatology: Some dermatologists specialize in pediatric dermatology, focusing on skin conditions affecting infants, children, and adolescents.

8. Dermatopathology: Dermatologists often work with dermatopathologists who analyze skin biopsies and tissue samples to aid in accurate diagnosis.

9. Phototherapy: Dermatologists may use light therapy (phototherapy) to treat certain skin conditions, such as psoriasis and vitiligo.

10. Skin Care Advice: They provide patients with personalized skincare recommendations to maintain healthy skin and prevent future skin problems.

11. Patient Education: Dermatologists educate patients about their skin conditions, treatment options, and how to protect their skin from harmful environmental factors, like UV radiation and pollution.

Dermatology is an ever-evolving field with ongoing research and advancements. It is important for individuals to seek professional advice if they have concerns about their skin, hair, or nails. Regular skin examinations and early intervention can play a significant role in maintaining skin health and preventing potential complications.

Skin Disorders and Dermatologic Conditions

Dermatologic conditions encompass a wide range of skin disorders, each with unique symptoms and treatments. Here are some common skin disorders and dermatologic conditions:

1. Acne: A skin condition characterized by pimples, blackheads, whiteheads, and sometimes deeper cysts. It often affects the face, chest, shoulders, and back.

2. Eczema (Atopic Dermatitis): A chronic inflammatory skin condition causing red, itchy, and irritated patches. It is common in children but can affect individuals of all ages.

3. Psoriasis: An autoimmune disorder that leads to the rapid buildup of skin cells, resulting in thick, red, and scaly patches on the skin. Psoriasis can affect any part of the body.

4. Rosacea: A chronic skin condition that causes redness, flushing, and the appearance of small, visible blood vessels on the face.

5. Dermatitis: A general term for inflammation of the skin, including contact dermatitis (caused by irritants or allergens) and seborrheic dermatitis (characterized by red, scaly patches on the scalp and face).

6. Hives (Urticaria): Raised, itchy welts on the skin that occur as an allergic reaction to various triggers, such as certain foods, medications, or insect stings.

7. Fungal Infections: These include athlete's foot, ringworm, and yeast infections, which can affect the

skin, nails, and hair.

8. Vitiligo: A condition that causes the loss of skin color in patches, resulting in white or depigmented areas on the skin.

9. Melasma: A common skin condition characterized by brown or gray-brown patches, often occurring on the face.

10.   Warts: Small, rough growths caused by the human papillomavirus (HPV) that can appear on various parts of the body.

11.   Impetigo: A highly contagious bacterial skin infection causing red sores that can break open, ooze, and form a yellow-brown crust.

12.   Cold Sores (Herpes Simplex Virus): Painful blisters that typically appear around the mouth, caused by the herpes simplex virus.

13.   Cellulitis: A bacterial skin infection that can cause redness, swelling, warmth, and tenderness of the skin.

14.   Skin Cancer: Various types of skin cancer, such as basal cell carcinoma, squamous cell carcinoma, and melanoma, can arise due to the uncontrolled growth of abnormal skin cells.

It is essential to consult a dermatologist for proper diagnosis and treatment if you suspect or experience any skin-related issues. Dermatologists can provide personalized care and recommend appropriate therapies to manage and improve various dermatologic conditions. Regular skin check-ups and preventive measures, such as wearing sunscreen and protective clothing, are essential for maintaining skin health and detecting potential skin cancer early.

Dermatologic Procedures and Cosmetic Interventions

Dermatologic procedures and cosmetic interventions are commonly performed by dermatologists to address various skin concerns and improve the appearance of the skin. Some of the most common procedures and interventions include:

1. Chemical Peels: A chemical solution is applied to the skin, causing it to exfoliate and peel off. This procedure helps improve skin texture, reduce fine lines, and treat certain types of acne and pigmentation issues.
2. Botox Injections: Botox is a neurotoxin that temporarily paralyzes muscles, reducing the appearance of wrinkles and fine lines on the face.
3. Dermal Fillers: Injectable fillers, such as hyaluronic acid, are used to add volume to areas of the face, improving wrinkles, sagging skin, and facial contours.
4. Laser Therapy: Various laser treatments are available for skin resurfacing, hair removal, pigmentation issues, and scar reduction.
5. Microdermabrasion: A non-invasive procedure that exfoliates the skin, helping to improve skin texture and reduce the appearance of fine lines and mild scars.
6. Cryotherapy: Liquid nitrogen is used to freeze and remove abnormal skin cells, such as warts and precancerous lesions.
7. Sclerotherapy: A treatment for spider and varicose veins, where a solution is injected directly into the affected veins, causing them to collapse and fade.

8. Dermabrasion: A more aggressive form of skin resurfacing, using a rotating instrument to remove the top layers of the skin, beneficial for scar reduction and skin rejuvenation.

9. Laser Hair Removal: Utilizing laser technology to target hair follicles, reducing hair growth in specific areas of the body.

10. Platelet-Rich Plasma (PRP) Therapy: A technique where a patient's own blood is used to stimulate collagen production and improve skin texture and elasticity.

11. Kybella: An injectable treatment used to reduce submental fat (double chin) by destroying fat cells.

12. Photodynamic Therapy: Combining a photosensitizing agent and light to treat certain skin conditions, such as acne and pre-cancerous lesions.

13. Liposuction: A surgical procedure used to remove excess fat from specific areas of the body.

14. Tattoo Removal: Using laser technology to break down tattoo pigments and eliminate unwanted tattoos.

It is crucial to consult a qualified and experienced dermatologist before undergoing any cosmetic procedures. A dermatologist can evaluate your specific skin concerns and recommend the most appropriate treatments for your needs, ensuring safe and effective results. Additionally, it is essential to have realistic expectations and understand potential risks associated with each procedure.

Dermatopathology and Biopsies

Dermatopathology is a specialized field of pathology that focuses on diagnosing skin diseases and disorders by examining skin tissue samples obtained through biopsies. Dermatopathologists are medical doctors who have completed additional training in both dermatology and pathology. They play a crucial role in accurately diagnosing skin conditions, as many skin diseases have similar clinical appearances but different underlying histological features.

Here is an overview of the process of dermatopathology and skin biopsies:

1. Skin Biopsy: When a dermatologist suspects a skin condition that requires further evaluation, they may perform a skin biopsy. During this procedure, a small sample of skin tissue is taken from the affected area, usually under local anesthesia.

2. Processing the Tissue: The skin tissue sample is sent to a laboratory, where it is processed and embedded in paraffin wax. This process allows the tissue to be thinly sliced and mounted on glass slides for microscopic examination.

3. Microscopic Examination: The dermatopathologist examines the stained tissue sections under a microscope to analyze the cellular and tissue changes. They look for specific patterns, cell types, and other characteristics that help in making an accurate diagnosis.

4. Diagnosis: Based on the microscopic findings and clinical information provided by the referring

dermatologist, the dermatopathologist provides a definitive diagnosis or a list of possible diagnoses. The final diagnosis guides the appropriate treatment and management of the skin condition.

5. Communication with the Dermatologist: The dermatopathologist communicates the results of the biopsy and diagnosis to the referring dermatologist, who then discusses the findings with the patient and develops a treatment plan.

Dermatopathology is essential in diagnosing various skin conditions, including inflammatory skin diseases, infections, benign growths, precancerous lesions, and skin cancers. The combination of clinical evaluation by the dermatologist and pathological assessment by the dermatopathologist ensures accurate diagnoses and appropriate patient care.

It is crucial to seek care from qualified and experienced dermatologists and dermatopathologists for any skin concerns or conditions. Early and accurate diagnosis plays a significant role in achieving successful treatment outcomes for skin diseases and disorders.

Epidemiology

Epidemiology is the branch of medical science that focuses on the study of the distribution, determinants, and frequency of diseases and health-related conditions in human populations. It plays a crucial role in public health by providing valuable information about the occurrence and patterns of diseases, which helps in identifying risk factors, developing preventive strategies, and improving overall health outcomes.

Key Concepts in Epidemiology:

1. Disease Occurrence: Epidemiologists study the occurrence of diseases and health conditions in populations. They collect data on the number of cases, the frequency of occurrence (incidence and prevalence), and trends over time.
2. Risk Factors: Epidemiologists identify risk factors that are associated with the development of specific diseases. These risk factors can be behavioral, environmental, genetic, or related to the individual's physiology or lifestyle.
3. Study Designs: Various study designs are used in epidemiology to investigate associations between risk factors and diseases. Common study designs include observational studies (e.g., cohort studies, case-control studies) and experimental studies (e.g., clinical trials).
4. Causality: Epidemiologists study the causal relationships between risk factors and diseases. Establishing causality involves demonstrating temporal relationships, biological plausibility, and consistency of findings across different studies.

5. Surveillance: Epidemiologists participate in disease surveillance, which involves the ongoing monitoring of disease occurrence and trends to detect outbreaks, track disease patterns, and inform public health interventions.

6. Outbreak Investigation: When disease outbreaks occur, epidemiologists play a critical role in investigating the source and transmission of the disease to control its spread and prevent further cases.

7. Public Health Interventions: Epidemiological findings contribute to the development of public health interventions and policies aimed at promoting health and preventing diseases in populations.

8. Data Analysis: Epidemiologists use statistical methods to analyze data and draw conclusions about disease patterns and associations between risk factors and health outcomes.

Epidemiology is used in various fields, including infectious disease control, chronic disease prevention, maternal and child health, environmental health, and occupational health. It is a key discipline in understanding the health status of populations and informing evidence-based decision-making in public health practice and policy.

Principles of Epidemiology and Disease Surveillance

Principles of Epidemiology:

1. Distribution: Epidemiology examines the distribution of diseases or health-related conditions across populations, including the frequency and patterns of occurrence. This involves studying factors such as age, gender, geographical location, and socio-economic status.

2. Determinants: Epidemiology identifies and investigates the determinants or risk factors that influence the occurrence of diseases. These determinants can be biological, behavioral, environmental, or social in nature.

3. Population Perspective: Epidemiology focuses on the health of populations rather than individual cases. It examines the health status and health outcomes of entire communities, regions, or countries.

4. Causation: Epidemiological studies aim to establish causal relationships between risk factors and diseases. This involves demonstrating a temporal relationship, dose-response association, biological plausibility, and consistency of findings across different studies.

5. Prevention: The primary goal of epidemiology is to inform prevention strategies and interventions. By identifying risk factors and understanding disease patterns, epidemiologists can recommend effective preventive measures.

6. Study Designs: Epidemiological research uses various study designs, including observational studies (cohort studies, case-control studies, cross-sectional studies) and experimental studies (randomized controlled trials). Each design has its strengths and limitations in addressing different research questions.

Disease Surveillance:

1. Definition: Disease surveillance involves the systematic collection, analysis, and interpretation of health-related data to track the occurrence and distribution of diseases or health conditions in a population.

2. Early Detection: Surveillance systems help in early detection of outbreaks or unusual health events. This allows for prompt response and control measures to prevent further spread.

3. Monitoring Trends: Disease surveillance monitors disease trends over time, which aids in identifying changes in disease incidence or prevalence, and provides valuable data for public health planning.

4. Evaluation of Control Measures: Surveillance data allows for the evaluation of the effectiveness of public health interventions and control measures in reducing disease burden.

5. Data Sources: Surveillance data can come from various sources, such as healthcare facilities, laboratories, electronic health records, public health agencies, and reporting systems.

6. Notifiable Diseases: Certain diseases are legally required to be reported to public health authorities, and disease surveillance systems play a crucial role in tracking these notifiable diseases.

7. Integration: Modern disease surveillance systems often use electronic health records and advanced data

analytics to improve data collection, integration, and analysis for timely and accurate reporting.

Both principles of epidemiology and disease surveillance are integral components of public health practice. They help in understanding the burden of diseases, identifying at-risk populations, developing targeted interventions, and assessing the impact of public health programs.

Outbreak Investigations and Public Health Interventions

Outbreak Investigations:

1. Definition: Outbreak investigations are systematic efforts to identify the cause and source of a sudden increase in the occurrence of a particular disease or health-related event within a specific population or geographic area.
2. Surveillance Systems: Early detection and reporting through disease surveillance systems are critical for initiating outbreak investigations. Surveillance data may indicate unusual trends or patterns that require further investigation.
3. Case Definition: Establishing a clear case definition is essential to determine which individuals are considered part of the outbreak and which are not. The case definition outlines specific criteria for inclusion based on clinical and epidemiological characteristics.
4. Case Finding: Once the case definition is established, investigators actively search for and identify additional cases to build a complete picture of the outbreak.
5. Case Investigation: Individual case investigations involve collecting detailed information about each case, including demographic data, symptoms, potential exposures, and other relevant factors.
6. Analytical Studies: Outbreak investigations may involve analytical studies, such as cohort studies or

case-control studies, to identify risk factors associated with the outbreak.

7. Source Identification: Investigators work to identify the source of the outbreak, which may be contaminated food, water, or other environmental exposures.

Public Health Interventions:

1. Control Measures: Public health interventions are implemented to control and contain outbreaks. These measures may include isolation and quarantine of affected individuals, treatment, and contact tracing.

2. Communication and Education: Effective communication with the public and healthcare professionals is crucial during an outbreak. Public health authorities provide timely and accurate information to raise awareness and ensure appropriate actions are taken.

3. Environmental Interventions: In outbreaks involving environmental exposures, public health interventions may include testing and cleaning of water sources, food recalls, or environmental decontamination.

4. Vaccination Campaigns: Vaccination is a powerful tool in preventing and controlling infectious disease outbreaks. Public health agencies may implement vaccination campaigns to protect susceptible populations.

5. Travel Restrictions: During outbreaks with international implications, travel restrictions may be imposed to prevent the spread of the disease to other regions or countries.

6. Surveillance Enhancement: In response to outbreaks, surveillance systems may be enhanced to increase monitoring and reporting of cases.

7. Evaluation and Monitoring: Public health

interventions are continuously evaluated to assess their effectiveness and adjust strategies as needed.

Outbreak investigations and public health interventions are essential components of disease control and prevention. Rapid and efficient responses can help contain outbreaks, reduce morbidity and mortality, and protect public health. Effective coordination between local, national, and international health authorities is crucial for managing outbreaks that may have broader implications.

Evidence-based Medicine and Data Analysis

Evidence-based Medicine (EBM) and Data Analysis:

Evidence-based medicine is an approach to clinical practice that involves integrating the best available evidence from research studies with clinical expertise and patient values to make informed decisions about patient care. Data analysis plays a crucial role in generating and interpreting the evidence used in evidence-based medicine. Here are key points about evidence-based medicine and its reliance on data analysis:

1. Evidence Hierarchy: Evidence-based medicine follows a hierarchy of evidence that ranks research studies based on their methodological rigor and potential for bias. Systematic reviews and meta-analyses of randomized controlled trials (RCTs) are considered the highest level of evidence, followed by RCTs, cohort studies, case-control studies, case series, and expert opinion.

2. Clinical Questions: In evidence-based medicine, clinical questions are formulated using the PICO framework (Population, Intervention, Comparison, Outcome). This structured approach helps in defining the specific question for which evidence is sought.

3. Literature Search: To gather evidence, systematic literature searches are performed in databases such as PubMed, Embase, and Cochrane Library. Data analysis in this stage involves screening and selecting relevant

studies based on predefined inclusion and exclusion criteria.

4. Critical Appraisal: Data analysis in evidence-based medicine involves critically appraising the selected studies to assess their methodological quality, potential biases, and generalizability of results.

5. Meta-Analysis: Meta-analysis is a statistical technique used to combine the results of multiple studies, providing a more robust estimate of the treatment effect. Data analysis in meta-analysis involves pooling data from individual studies, calculating effect sizes, and assessing heterogeneity among studies.

6. Clinical Guidelines: Evidence-based medicine forms the basis for developing clinical practice guidelines, which provide recommendations for healthcare professionals based on the best available evidence.

7. Clinical Decision Support: Data analysis plays a role in developing clinical decision support tools that aid healthcare providers in making evidence-based decisions at the point of care.

8. Continuous Learning: Evidence-based medicine emphasizes the importance of continuous learning and keeping up-to-date with new research findings. Data analysis is integral to staying informed about the latest evidence and its impact on patient care.

9. Limitations of Evidence: Evidence-based medicine acknowledges that not all clinical questions can be answered with high-quality evidence. In such cases, clinical judgment and patient preferences play a significant role in decision-making.

10. Patient-Centered Care: Evidence-based medicine recognizes the importance of incorporating patient preferences and values into clinical decision-making, ensuring that care is tailored to individual patients.

Data analysis is a fundamental component of evidence-based medicine, enabling healthcare professionals to translate research findings into meaningful and applicable information for patient care. By combining the best available evidence with clinical expertise and patient values, evidence-based medicine promotes high-quality, patient-centered care.

Geriatrics

Geriatrics is a medical specialty focused on the health and care of older adults. It involves the prevention, diagnosis, and treatment of age-related conditions and the management of complex health issues that are common in elderly individuals. Here are some key aspects of geriatrics:

1. Age Consideration: Geriatrics specifically addresses the unique health needs of older adults, typically focusing on individuals aged 65 and above. As people age, they become more susceptible to various medical conditions and require specialized care.

2. Multidimensional Approach: Geriatric care takes a holistic and multidimensional approach, considering not only medical conditions but also social, psychological, and functional aspects of aging.

3. Common Geriatric Conditions: Geriatricians often encounter age-related conditions such as arthritis, osteoporosis, cardiovascular diseases, dementia, depression, falls, and urinary incontinence.

4. Comprehensive Geriatric Assessment: Comprehensive geriatric assessment (CGA) is a core aspect of geriatric care. It involves a thorough evaluation of an older adult's medical, cognitive, functional, social, and environmental aspects to develop an individualized care plan.

5. Polypharmacy Management: Older adults may be taking multiple medications for various health conditions. Geriatric specialists emphasize the importance of optimizing medication regimens,

minimizing polypharmacy, and reducing potential drug interactions.

6. Functional Assessment: Geriatrics places significant emphasis on assessing an older adult's functional abilities, including mobility, activities of daily living (ADLs), and instrumental activities of daily living (IADLs).

7. Preventive Care: Geriatric care focuses on preventive measures to maintain and improve the health of older adults, including vaccinations, fall prevention strategies, and early detection of age-related diseases.

8. Palliative Care and End-of-Life Issues: Geriatricians are skilled in providing palliative care, which aims to improve the quality of life for older adults with serious illnesses. They also address end-of-life issues and assist patients and families in making appropriate care decisions.

9. Caregiver Support: Geriatrics involves providing support and resources to family caregivers who play a vital role in the care of older adults.

10. Interdisciplinary Approach: Geriatric care often involves a team of healthcare professionals, including geriatricians, nurses, social workers, physical therapists, occupational therapists, and others, who collaborate to provide comprehensive care.

11. Aging in Place: Geriatrics promotes the concept of "aging in place," allowing older adults to remain in their homes and communities with the necessary support and services.

12. Health Promotion: Geriatric care includes health promotion strategies to encourage healthy lifestyle choices and preventive behaviors in older adults.

Geriatrics plays a crucial role in addressing the diverse health needs of the aging population and promoting healthy aging. It aims to improve the quality of life, functional independence, and overall well-being of older adults through specialized and personalized care.

Aging and Age-Related Health Concerns

Aging is a natural and inevitable process that affects all living organisms, including humans. As people age, their bodies undergo various physical, physiological, and psychological changes, which can lead to an increased risk of certain health concerns. While aging is a normal part of life, it is essential to be aware of age-related health issues to promote healthy aging and early detection of potential problems. Here are some common age-related health concerns:

1. Cardiovascular Diseases: As people age, the risk of cardiovascular diseases, such as hypertension, heart disease, and stroke, increases. Maintaining a healthy lifestyle and managing risk factors like high blood pressure, cholesterol levels, and diabetes can help prevent or delay the onset of these conditions.

2. Osteoporosis: Aging can lead to a loss of bone density, making older adults more susceptible to fractures and osteoporosis. Adequate calcium and vitamin D intake, regular weight-bearing exercises, and falls prevention measures are crucial for maintaining bone health.

3. Arthritis: Arthritis is a common age-related condition characterized by joint pain, stiffness, and inflammation. Gentle exercises, physical therapy, and medication management can help alleviate symptoms and improve joint function.

4. Cognitive Decline and Dementia: Cognitive decline is a normal part of aging, but severe cognitive impairment,

such as dementia (e.g., Alzheimer's disease), can significantly impact daily functioning. Engaging in mentally stimulating activities and adopting a brain-healthy lifestyle may help support cognitive function.

5. Vision and Hearing Loss: Age-related changes in the eyes and ears can lead to vision and hearing problems. Regular eye exams and hearing tests are essential for early detection and appropriate interventions.

6. Falls and Fractures: Aging can affect balance and coordination, increasing the risk of falls and fractures. Exercise programs that improve strength and balance, along with home safety measures, can help reduce fall-related injuries.

7. Urinary Incontinence: Bladder control issues, such as urinary incontinence, can become more prevalent with age. Pelvic floor exercises and lifestyle modifications can be effective in managing this condition.

8. Sleep Problems: Sleep patterns may change with age, leading to insomnia or other sleep disorders. Establishing good sleep habits and addressing underlying health issues can promote better sleep.

9. Depression and Mental Health: Older adults may face challenges related to loss, loneliness, or changes in life circumstances, which can contribute to depression and mental health concerns. Seeking support and maintaining social connections are essential for mental well-being.

10. Chronic Diseases: Older adults are more likely to have chronic health conditions, such as diabetes, chronic obstructive pulmonary disease (COPD), and kidney disease. Proper management and adherence to medical treatments are crucial for disease control.

While aging is associated with certain health challenges,

maintaining a healthy lifestyle, regular medical check-ups, and preventive care can significantly improve the quality of life in older adults. It's essential for older individuals and their caregivers to be proactive in addressing age-related health concerns and seeking appropriate medical attention when needed.

Geriatric Assessment and Multidimensional Care

Geriatric assessment is a comprehensive evaluation of an older adult's overall health and functional status. It goes beyond the traditional medical evaluation and considers multiple dimensions of a person's well-being, including physical, psychological, social, and functional aspects. The goal of geriatric assessment is to develop a tailored care plan that addresses the specific needs and challenges faced by older individuals to promote optimal health and quality of life.

Components of Geriatric Assessment:

1. Medical History: A detailed review of the person's medical history, including past illnesses, medications, surgeries, and chronic conditions.
2. Physical Examination: A thorough examination to assess physical health, mobility, sensory functions, and any signs of age-related changes.
3. Cognitive Function: Assessment of cognitive abilities, memory, attention, and executive functions to identify any cognitive impairment or dementia.
4. Functional Status: Evaluation of the person's ability to perform daily activities, such as bathing, dressing, eating, and mobility.
5. Mental Health: Screening for depression, anxiety, and other mental health issues that can be common in older adults.
6. Social and Environmental Factors: An examination of

the person's social support network, living situation, and access to community resources.

7. Nutritional Status: Assessment of nutritional intake and potential malnutrition or dietary deficiencies.

8. Medication Review: A comprehensive review of medications to ensure appropriate use and minimize potential drug interactions.

9. Assessment of Fall Risk: Identification of factors that may increase the risk of falls, with appropriate interventions to reduce fall-related injuries.

Benefits of Geriatric Assessment:

1. Personalized Care: The assessment helps healthcare providers develop individualized care plans that address specific needs and challenges faced by older adults.

2. Early Detection: It can help identify health problems, cognitive changes, or functional limitations at an early stage, leading to timely intervention.

3. Comprehensive Approach: Geriatric assessment considers the multiple dimensions of health, ensuring a holistic approach to care.

4. Improved Communication: It facilitates better communication among healthcare providers, older individuals, and their caregivers, leading to more informed decision-making.

5. Enhanced Quality of Life: By addressing physical, emotional, and social needs, geriatric assessment aims to improve the overall quality of life for older adults.

Multidimensional Care:

Multidimensional care involves a collaborative and interdisciplinary approach to managing the health and well-being of older adults. It recognizes that addressing the complex needs of older individuals often requires input from various healthcare professionals, caregivers, and social services. The multidimensional care team may include primary care physicians, geriatric specialists, nurses, physical and occupational therapists, social workers, psychologists, and nutritionists.

The team works together to develop a comprehensive care plan that incorporates the findings of the geriatric assessment and addresses all aspects of the person's health. Regular communication among team members ensures continuity of care and allows for adjustments to the care plan as needed.

Multidimensional care also emphasizes shared decision-making, involving the older adult and their family in the decision-making process regarding their health and well-being.

Overall, geriatric assessment and multidimensional care play a crucial role in meeting the unique healthcare needs of older adults, promoting healthy aging, and enhancing their quality of life.

Palliative Care and End-of-Life Considerations

Palliative care is a specialized medical approach focused on improving the quality of life for individuals facing serious illnesses or life-limiting conditions. Its primary goal is to provide relief from physical, emotional, and psychological symptoms, while also addressing the spiritual and social needs of patients and their families. Palliative care can be provided at any stage of a serious illness, alongside curative treatments or as the main focus of care.

Key Aspects of Palliative Care:

1. Symptom Management: Palliative care aims to alleviate pain, manage symptoms like nausea, fatigue, and breathlessness, and improve overall comfort for patients.

2. Emotional and Psychological Support: Palliative care teams provide emotional and psychological support to both patients and their families, helping them cope with the challenges of serious illness and end-of-life issues.

3. Communication and Shared Decision-making: Palliative care involves open and honest communication between healthcare providers, patients, and families to ensure informed decision-making about treatment options and goals of care.

4. Holistic Approach: Palliative care takes a holistic approach, considering not only physical symptoms

but also the psychosocial, spiritual, and cultural needs of patients and their families.

5. Advance Care Planning: Palliative care teams help patients and families discuss and document their healthcare preferences, including end-of-life care decisions, through advance care planning.

6. Continuity of Care: Palliative care aims to provide consistent and continuous care, involving a team of healthcare professionals working together to meet the patient's needs.

Palliative care can be provided in various settings, such as hospitals, hospices, long-term care facilities, or the patient's home, depending on the individual's needs and preferences.

End-of-Life Considerations:

As a part of palliative care, end-of-life considerations focus on supporting patients and their families during the final stages of life. It involves respecting the patient's choices, providing comfort and dignity, and ensuring that the patient's wishes are honored.

End-of-life considerations may include:

1. Hospice Care: Hospice care is a specific type of palliative care provided for individuals with a life expectancy of six months or less. It focuses on providing comfort and support during the end of life, often in a home or hospice facility.

2. Pain and Symptom Management: During end-of-life care, ensuring effective pain and symptom management is crucial to providing comfort and improving the quality of life for the patient.

3. Emotional and Spiritual Support: End-of-life care involves providing emotional and spiritual support to both patients and their families, helping them navigate the emotional challenges of this phase.

4. Family Involvement: Supporting the patient's family in understanding and coping with the dying process is an essential aspect of end-of-life care.
5. Respect for Cultural and Spiritual Beliefs: End-of-life care should be respectful of the patient's cultural and spiritual beliefs, ensuring that their wishes are honored.
6. Bereavement Support: Bereavement support is provided to the family after the patient's death, helping them cope with grief and loss.

Overall, palliative care and end-of-life considerations aim to enhance the quality of life for patients facing serious illnesses, and to ensure that their wishes and preferences are respected during their final stages of life.

Hepatology

Hepatology is a branch of medicine focused on the study, diagnosis, and treatment of liver-related diseases and disorders. The liver is a vital organ responsible for various functions, including detoxification, metabolism, and production of important proteins. Hepatologists are medical specialists who have expertise in managing liver diseases and work closely with gastroenterologists, internists, and other healthcare professionals to provide comprehensive care for patients with liver conditions.

Key Aspects of Hepatology:

1. Liver Diseases: Hepatologists diagnose and treat a wide range of liver diseases, including viral hepatitis (such as hepatitis B and C), fatty liver disease, alcoholic liver disease, autoimmune liver diseases (like autoimmune hepatitis and primary biliary cirrhosis), liver cirrhosis, liver cancer (hepatocellular carcinoma), and various genetic liver disorders.

2. Liver Function Testing: Hepatologists use various laboratory tests to assess liver function and diagnose liver diseases. Common tests include liver enzymes (ALT, AST, ALP), bilirubin levels, albumin, and clotting factors.

3. Imaging Studies: Hepatologists may order imaging studies such as ultrasound, CT scans, or MRI to evaluate the liver's size, structure, and identify any abnormalities or liver tumors.

4. Liver Biopsy: In certain cases, a liver biopsy may be recommended to obtain a tissue sample from the liver

for a more accurate diagnosis and assessment of liver damage.

5. Treatment and Management: Treatment strategies for liver diseases vary depending on the underlying condition. Hepatologists may prescribe antiviral medications for viral hepatitis, recommend lifestyle changes for fatty liver disease, manage autoimmune liver diseases with immunosuppressive drugs, or provide other targeted therapies based on the specific liver condition.

6. Liver Transplantation: In cases of advanced liver disease or liver failure, hepatologists may be involved in the evaluation, preparation, and follow-up care of patients undergoing liver transplantation.

7. Multidisciplinary Approach: Hepatology often involves collaboration with other medical specialties, such as gastroenterology, oncology, radiology, and transplant surgery, to provide comprehensive care for patients with complex liver conditions.

Hepatology plays a crucial role in diagnosing and managing liver diseases, improving patient outcomes, and preventing complications associated with liver disorders. Regular screenings, early detection, and proper management are essential for maintaining liver health and preventing serious liver-related complications.

Liver Function and Hepatic Diseases

The liver is a vital organ responsible for performing numerous essential functions that are crucial for maintaining overall health. Some of the key functions of the liver include:

1. Metabolism: The liver plays a central role in the metabolism of carbohydrates, proteins, and fats. It stores and releases glucose as needed, synthesizes proteins, and converts excess nutrients into storage forms.
2. Detoxification: The liver detoxifies the body by processing and eliminating various harmful substances, including drugs, alcohol, and metabolic waste products.
3. Bile Production: The liver produces bile, a fluid that aids in the digestion and absorption of fats in the small intestine.
4. Storage of Vitamins and Minerals: The liver stores essential vitamins (A, D, E, and K) and minerals (such as iron and copper) for future use.

Given the liver's critical functions, any disruption or damage to the organ can lead to hepatic diseases. Some common liver diseases and conditions include:

1. Hepatitis: Hepatitis refers to inflammation of the liver, which can be caused by viral infections (hepatitis A, B, C, D, and E) or non-viral factors like alcohol abuse, autoimmune diseases, or certain medications.
2. Fatty Liver Disease: Fatty liver disease is characterized by an accumulation of fat within the liver cells. It

can occur due to alcohol consumption (alcoholic fatty liver disease) or non-alcoholic factors, such as obesity, insulin resistance, and metabolic syndrome (non-alcoholic fatty liver disease or NAFLD).

3. Cirrhosis: Cirrhosis is the advanced stage of liver scarring and fibrosis. It is often a result of long-term liver damage from chronic hepatitis, alcohol abuse, or other liver diseases.

4. Liver Cancer: Primary liver cancer, or hepatocellular carcinoma, is a type of cancer that originates in the liver. It is commonly associated with underlying liver diseases, such as chronic hepatitis or cirrhosis.

5. Liver Failure: Liver failure occurs when the liver's ability to function is severely compromised, leading to life-threatening complications.

6. Autoimmune Liver Diseases: Conditions like autoimmune hepatitis, primary biliary cholangitis (PBC), and primary sclerosing cholangitis (PSC) are characterized by the body's immune system mistakenly attacking the liver.

Regular medical check-ups and screenings are essential to detect liver diseases early and initiate timely treatment. Preventive measures, such as maintaining a healthy lifestyle, avoiding excessive alcohol consumption, and getting vaccinated against hepatitis, can help protect the liver and promote overall liver health. Hepatology specialists play a critical role in diagnosing and managing liver diseases and guiding patients toward better liver health outcomes.

Diagnosis and Management of Liver Disorders

The diagnosis and management of liver disorders involve a comprehensive approach that includes clinical evaluation, laboratory tests, imaging studies, and, in some cases, liver biopsies. Here is an overview of the steps involved in diagnosing and managing liver disorders:

1. Clinical Evaluation: The process begins with a thorough medical history and physical examination. The healthcare provider will inquire about symptoms, risk factors, family history, and lifestyle habits (such as alcohol consumption and drug use).
2. Blood Tests: Blood tests are essential for assessing liver function and detecting abnormalities. Common liver function tests include liver enzymes (AST, ALT, ALP, GGT), bilirubin, albumin, and INR (international normalized ratio).
3. Imaging Studies: Imaging techniques, such as ultrasound, CT scan, or MRI, may be used to evaluate the liver's structure and detect any abnormalities, such as tumors or cirrhosis.
4. Viral Hepatitis Testing: Specific blood tests are used to identify viral hepatitis infections (hepatitis A, B, C, D, and E).
5. Liver Biopsy: In some cases, a liver biopsy may be performed to obtain a small tissue sample from the liver for microscopic examination. It helps diagnose liver diseases like hepatitis, cirrhosis, and liver cancer.

6. Non-Invasive Tests: Non-invasive methods, such as FibroScan or FibroTest, are used to assess liver fibrosis without the need for a liver biopsy.

Once the diagnosis is confirmed, the management of liver disorders depends on the specific condition and its severity. Treatment options may include:

1. Lifestyle Modifications: For non-alcoholic fatty liver disease (NAFLD), lifestyle changes such as weight loss, regular exercise, and a healthy diet can improve liver health.
2. Antiviral Therapy: Antiviral medications are used to treat chronic viral hepatitis (e.g., hepatitis B and C) to suppress viral replication and reduce liver inflammation.
3. Medications: Medications may be prescribed to manage symptoms and slow the progression of certain liver diseases.
4. Liver Transplantation: For severe liver diseases such as cirrhosis or liver failure, a liver transplant may be considered as a last resort when other treatments are ineffective.
5. Management of Underlying Conditions: Treatment of underlying conditions, such as autoimmune diseases or metabolic disorders, is essential to improve liver function.
6. Regular Follow-up: Regular follow-up visits with a hepatologist or gastroenterologist are crucial to monitor liver function and adjust the treatment plan as needed.

It's important to note that early diagnosis and timely intervention play a significant role in the successful management of liver disorders. Individuals with known liver conditions should work closely with their healthcare providers to ensure proper monitoring and adherence to the recommended treatment plan. Additionally, avoiding alcohol abuse and adopting a healthy lifestyle can contribute to better liver health and overall well-being.

Liver Transplantation and Post-transplant Care

Liver transplantation is a surgical procedure where a diseased or damaged liver is replaced with a healthy liver from a donor. It is considered a life-saving treatment for end-stage liver disease and certain liver cancers. After liver transplantation, post-transplant care is essential to ensure a successful outcome and long-term survival. Here's an overview of the process and post-transplant care:

1. Pre-Transplant Evaluation: Before undergoing liver transplantation, candidates are thoroughly evaluated to assess their suitability for the procedure. The evaluation includes medical history, physical examination, blood tests, imaging studies, and psychological evaluation. The patient's overall health and ability to withstand the surgery and recovery process are assessed.

2. Waiting List: Patients who are deemed eligible for liver transplantation are placed on a waiting list for a donor liver. The waiting time depends on factors such as the severity of the liver disease, blood type, and availability of donor organs.

3. Transplant Surgery: Once a suitable donor liver becomes available, the transplant surgery is performed. During the procedure, the damaged liver is removed, and the donor liver is implanted. The surgery can take several hours, and the patient is typically placed under general anesthesia.

4. Post-Transplant Recovery: After the surgery, the patient is closely monitored in the intensive care unit (ICU) for a period before being transferred to a regular hospital room. The recovery process may vary depending on the individual's overall health and the complexity of the surgery.

5. Immunosuppression: To prevent the body from rejecting the transplanted liver, patients are prescribed immunosuppressive medications. These drugs suppress the immune system's response, reducing the risk of organ rejection. Adherence to the prescribed immunosuppressive regimen is crucial to ensure the long-term success of the transplant.

6. Post-Transplant Follow-up: After discharge from the hospital, patients will have frequent follow-up visits with their transplant team. These visits include regular blood tests, imaging studies, and monitoring of liver function to detect any signs of rejection or complications.

7. Rehabilitation and Lifestyle Changes: After liver transplantation, patients may require physical therapy and rehabilitation to regain strength and mobility. Lifestyle changes, such as maintaining a healthy diet, avoiding alcohol and smoking, and staying physically active, are essential for the well-being of the transplanted liver.

8. Infection Prevention: Due to the suppressed immune system, transplant recipients are at a higher risk of infections. It's crucial to take measures to prevent infections, such as practicing good hygiene, avoiding contact with sick individuals, and getting recommended vaccinations.

9. Emotional Support: Liver transplantation can be a life-altering experience for patients and their families. Emotional support and counseling may be beneficial to help cope with the challenges and adjustments after

the surgery.

10.   Long-term Care: Liver transplant recipients require lifelong medical follow-up and care. Regular monitoring of liver function, immunosuppressive medication adjustments, and screenings for potential complications are part of the long-term management.

It's important for liver transplant recipients to maintain open communication with their transplant team, adhere to medical recommendations, and promptly report any unusual symptoms or concerns. Following the prescribed post-transplant care plan is essential to ensure the success of the transplant and to enjoy improved quality of life after the procedure.

Obstetrics & Gynecology

Obstetrics and gynecology (OB/GYN) is a medical specialty that focuses on the health and well-being of women, particularly during pregnancy, childbirth, and the postpartum period. It also encompasses the diagnosis and treatment of various gynecological conditions throughout a woman's life. Here's an overview of obstetrics and gynecology:

1. Obstetrics: Obstetrics deals with the management of pregnancy, childbirth, and the postpartum period. Obstetricians are specialists who provide prenatal care, assist in labor and delivery, and offer postpartum care to both the mother and newborn. They monitor the health and development of the fetus during pregnancy and ensure a safe delivery.

2. Prenatal Care: Prenatal care involves regular medical check-ups and monitoring during pregnancy. Obstetricians track the baby's growth, screen for potential health issues, and provide guidance on proper nutrition, exercise, and overall well-being during pregnancy.

3. Labor and Delivery: Obstetricians are responsible for managing labor and delivery. They assist in vaginal deliveries and perform cesarean sections when necessary. Obstetricians work closely with labor and delivery nurses, anesthesiologists, and other healthcare providers to ensure a safe and positive birthing experience.

4. Postpartum Care: After childbirth, obstetricians continue to monitor the mother's recovery and

the newborn's health during the postpartum period. They address any postpartum concerns, provide breastfeeding support, and offer guidance on postpartum self-care.

5. Gynecology: Gynecology involves the diagnosis and treatment of conditions related to the female reproductive system, excluding pregnancy and childbirth. Gynecologists provide preventive care, medical management, and surgical interventions for various gynecological conditions.

6. Routine Gynecological Examinations: Gynecologists perform routine pelvic exams and Pap smears to screen for cervical cancer and other gynecological conditions. These exams are essential for maintaining women's reproductive health and detecting potential issues early on.

7. Management of Menstrual Disorders: Gynecologists diagnose and treat menstrual disorders such as irregular periods, heavy bleeding, and painful periods. They offer medical and surgical solutions to manage these conditions.

8. Contraception and Family Planning: Gynecologists provide counseling on contraception options and family planning. They can prescribe birth control methods suitable for each individual's needs and preferences.

9. Management of Menopause: Gynecologists offer support and management for women going through menopause, addressing symptoms such as hot flashes, mood changes, and vaginal dryness. They may recommend hormone replacement therapy or other treatments to alleviate symptoms.

10.   Gynecologic Surgeries: Gynecologists perform various surgical procedures, including hysterectomy (removal of the uterus), myomectomy (removal of uterine fibroids), and laparoscopic

surgeries for gynecological conditions.

Obstetricians and gynecologists play a vital role in women's health and are advocates for their patients' overall well-being. They provide comprehensive care throughout a woman's life, from adolescence to menopause and beyond. Women are encouraged to have regular check-ups with their OB/GYN to promote optimal health and address any reproductive health concerns.

Maternal and Women's Health

Maternal and women's health focuses on the well-being of women during their reproductive years, including pregnancy, childbirth, and the postpartum period, as well as other gynecological and general health concerns throughout a woman's life. It encompasses various aspects of healthcare tailored to meet the unique needs of women. Here's an overview of maternal and women's health:

1. Preconception Care: Preconception care involves medical assessment and counseling before a woman becomes pregnant. It focuses on optimizing the woman's health to ensure a healthy pregnancy and baby. Preconception care may include lifestyle modifications, vaccination updates, and screening for health conditions that could affect pregnancy.

2. Prenatal Care: Prenatal care is crucial during pregnancy to monitor the health of both the mother and the developing baby. Regular prenatal check-ups include physical examinations, ultrasounds, and various tests to assess fetal development and identify any potential issues. Prenatal care also involves providing guidance on proper nutrition, exercise, and managing common pregnancy symptoms.

3. Labor and Delivery: Maternal health professionals, including obstetricians and midwives, provide care and support during labor and delivery. They assist with vaginal births and perform cesarean sections when necessary. The goal is to ensure a safe and positive birthing experience for both the mother and

the baby.

4. Postpartum Care: Postpartum care focuses on the mother's recovery after childbirth and the well-being of the newborn. Healthcare providers monitor the mother's physical and emotional health and provide support with breastfeeding, newborn care, and postpartum self-care.

5. Gynecological Care: Maternal and women's health encompasses routine gynecological exams and screenings to maintain reproductive health. These exams may include pelvic exams, Pap smears, breast exams, and other tests to detect gynecological issues and cancers early.

6. Family Planning and Contraception: Women's health services include counseling on family planning and contraception options. Healthcare providers help women choose birth control methods that align with their lifestyle and reproductive goals.

7. Menopause Management: Women's health professionals offer support and management for women going through menopause. They address symptoms such as hot flashes, mood changes, and bone health concerns. Menopause management may involve hormone replacement therapy and lifestyle adjustments.

8. Management of Gynecological Conditions: Maternal and women's health specialists diagnose and treat various gynecological conditions, including menstrual disorders, pelvic pain, and reproductive organ issues.

9. Women's Wellness: In addition to reproductive health, maternal and women's health emphasizes overall wellness and preventive care. It includes promoting healthy lifestyle choices, managing chronic conditions, and addressing mental health concerns.

Maternal and women's health aims to provide comprehensive care that addresses the unique needs and challenges women face throughout their lives. Healthcare providers in this field strive to empower women to make informed decisions about their health and support them in achieving optimal well-being at every stage of life. Regular check-ups and communication with healthcare professionals are essential for maintaining women's health and preventing or addressing any health issues that may arise.

Obstetric and Gynecologic Surgeries

Obstetric and gynecologic surgeries are specialized procedures performed on the female reproductive system. These surgeries are designed to diagnose and treat various conditions related to pregnancy, childbirth, and gynecological health. Some common obstetric and gynecologic surgeries include:

1. Cesarean Section (C-section): A cesarean section is a surgical procedure in which the baby is delivered through an incision made in the mother's abdomen and uterus. C-sections are performed when vaginal delivery is not safe or possible for the mother or baby.

2. Hysterectomy: A hysterectomy is the surgical removal of the uterus. It may be performed for various reasons, including uterine fibroids, endometriosis, cancer, chronic pelvic pain, or excessive bleeding that does not respond to other treatments.

3. Oophorectomy: An oophorectomy is the surgical removal of one or both ovaries. It may be done to treat ovarian cysts, endometriosis, or ovarian cancer.

4. Myomectomy: A myomectomy is the surgical removal of uterine fibroids while preserving the uterus. It is performed to alleviate symptoms such as heavy menstrual bleeding and pelvic pain.

5. Hysteroscopy: Hysteroscopy is a minimally invasive procedure in which a thin, lighted tube (hysteroscope) is inserted through the vagina into the uterus to examine the uterine lining and diagnose or treat conditions like polyps or fibroids.

6. Laparoscopy: Laparoscopy is a minimally invasive

VIKASH DABRIWAL

surgical technique in which a small camera is inserted through a small incision in the abdomen to visualize and operate on the pelvic organs, including the uterus, ovaries, and fallopian tubes.

7. Tubal Ligation: Tubal ligation, also known as female sterilization, is a surgical procedure to permanently prevent pregnancy by blocking or sealing the fallopian tubes.

8. Colposcopy: Colposcopy is a procedure in which a colposcope is used to examine the cervix, vagina, and vulva for abnormalities. It is often performed to follow up on abnormal Pap smear results or to diagnose cervical dysplasia or cancer.

9. Endometrial Ablation: Endometrial ablation is a procedure that destroys the uterine lining to reduce or stop menstrual bleeding. It is used for women with heavy menstrual periods who do not wish to undergo a hysterectomy.

10. Pelvic Organ Prolapse Repair: Pelvic organ prolapse occurs when the pelvic organs (such as the bladder, uterus, or rectum) descend or bulge into the vaginal canal. Surgical procedures can be performed to restore the organs to their normal position.

These are just a few examples of the various obstetric and gynecologic surgeries performed to address specific conditions affecting the female reproductive system. The choice of surgery depends on the individual's medical history, condition, and desired outcome. It is essential to consult with a qualified obstetrician-gynecologist to determine the most appropriate treatment plan for each patient's unique needs.

Fertility Treatments and Reproductive Medicine

Fertility treatments and reproductive medicine are medical interventions designed to assist individuals or couples who have difficulty conceiving a child naturally. These treatments aim to improve fertility, facilitate conception, and support successful pregnancies. Some common fertility treatments and reproductive medicine techniques include:

1. Ovulation Induction: This involves the use of medications, such as clomiphene citrate or gonadotropins, to stimulate the ovaries and induce ovulation in women who are not ovulating regularly or have irregular menstrual cycles.

2. Intrauterine Insemination (IUI): IUI is a procedure in which prepared sperm is placed directly into the woman's uterus during her fertile window to increase the chances of sperm reaching the egg.

3. In vitro Fertilization (IVF): IVF is a highly effective assisted reproductive technology where eggs are retrieved from the woman's ovaries and fertilized with sperm in a laboratory. The resulting embryos are then transferred back into the woman's uterus.

4. Intracytoplasmic Sperm Injection (ICSI): ICSI is a technique used in conjunction with IVF, where a single sperm is directly injected into an egg to facilitate fertilization, especially in cases of male infertility.

5. Assisted Hatching: Assisted hatching involves creating a small opening in the outer shell (zona pellucida) of

the embryo to aid in its implantation into the uterus during IVF.

6. Preimplantation Genetic Testing (PGT): PGT is performed on embryos before transfer to identify genetic abnormalities, chromosomal disorders, or specific genetic conditions.

7. Egg and Sperm Donation: Donor eggs or sperm may be used when one partner has fertility issues or same-sex couples seek to conceive.

8. Surrogacy: Surrogacy involves using a gestational carrier to carry and deliver a child for intended parents who cannot carry a pregnancy themselves.

9. Fertility Preservation: This involves freezing eggs, sperm, or embryos for future use, especially in cases where individuals are facing medical treatments that may affect fertility.

10. Reproductive Endocrinology: This specialized field of medicine deals with hormonal disorders affecting fertility and reproductive health.

Fertility treatments and reproductive medicine are continually evolving, offering hope and opportunities for individuals and couples facing infertility challenges. However, it is essential to work closely with a qualified reproductive specialist or fertility clinic to explore the most suitable options based on individual medical histories, needs, and preferences. These treatments require careful consideration, personalized care, and ongoing support to achieve the best possible outcomes.

Osteopathy

Osteopathy is a holistic and patient-centered approach to healthcare that focuses on the interrelationship between the body's structure and function. Osteopathic medicine emphasizes the body's inherent ability to heal itself and aims to promote health and well-being through the enhancement of the body's own healing mechanisms.

Key principles of osteopathy include:

1. The body is a unit: Osteopaths view the body as a unified whole, where all parts are interconnected and function together.
2. Structure and function are interrelated: The structure of the body, including bones, muscles, ligaments, and organs, influences its function, and vice versa.
3. The body's self-healing ability: Osteopaths believe that the body has an innate ability to heal and maintain health. Their role is to support and facilitate this natural healing process.
4. The importance of the musculoskeletal system: Osteopathy places significant emphasis on the musculoskeletal system, as it plays a crucial role in maintaining overall health and wellness.

Osteopathic physicians, also known as osteopaths or DOs (Doctors of Osteopathic Medicine), undergo rigorous medical training similar to allopathic (MD) physicians but with additional training in osteopathic manipulative treatment (OMT). OMT is a hands-on approach used by osteopathic physicians to diagnose and treat various musculoskeletal conditions, promote healing, and restore balance within the body.

Osteopathic treatment may include a range of manual techniques, such as gentle stretching, pressure, and manipulation of muscles and joints, to address musculoskeletal issues, improve circulation, and enhance nerve function. OMT is often used to alleviate pain, improve mobility, and support the body's natural healing processes.

Osteopathic medicine is used to treat a wide variety of conditions, including:

1. Musculoskeletal pain and injuries, such as back pain, neck pain, and joint pain.
2. Headaches and migraines.
3. Chronic pain conditions, such as fibromyalgia.
4. Postural imbalances and alignment issues.
5. Respiratory conditions, such as asthma and chronic obstructive pulmonary disease (COPD).
6. Digestive disorders, such as irritable bowel syndrome (IBS).
7. Women's health issues, including menstrual irregularities and pregnancy-related discomfort.
8. Sports-related injuries and performance enhancement.

In addition to OMT, osteopathic physicians also use traditional medical treatments, medications, and surgical interventions when necessary. They take a comprehensive and holistic approach to patient care, considering not only physical health but also lifestyle, nutrition, and emotional well-being.

Osteopathy is recognized as a complementary and alternative medicine (CAM) modality and is increasingly integrated into mainstream healthcare systems worldwide. Osteopathic physicians work in various healthcare settings, including private practices, hospitals, clinics, and academic institutions, collaborating with other healthcare professionals to provide comprehensive and patient-centered care.

Osteopathic Medicine and Holistic Approach to Patient Care

Osteopathic medicine is a unique branch of healthcare that emphasizes a holistic approach to patient care. Osteopathic physicians, also known as osteopaths or DOs (Doctors of Osteopathic Medicine), are medical doctors who have completed medical school and specialized training in osteopathic manipulative treatment (OMT). They use a whole-person approach to diagnosis, treatment, and prevention, considering not only the physical aspects of the patient but also their emotional, mental, and social well-being.

The key components of the holistic approach in osteopathic medicine include:

1. Focus on the Body's Structure and Function: Osteopaths believe that the body's structure (bones, muscles, ligaments, and organs) is closely related to its function. Structural imbalances can lead to health issues, and restoring balance through osteopathic manipulative treatment can facilitate healing and improve overall health.

2. Integration of Body Systems: Osteopathic physicians recognize that the body's systems are interconnected and work together. They consider how dysfunction in one system may affect others and aim to address the root causes of health problems rather than merely treating symptoms.

3. Emphasis on the Body's Innate Healing Ability:

Osteopaths believe in the body's inherent ability to heal itself. Their role is to support and enhance the body's natural healing mechanisms through various interventions, including OMT, lifestyle modifications, and appropriate medical treatments.

4. Patient-Centered Care: Osteopathic physicians view each patient as a unique individual with specific needs and circumstances. They take the time to listen to their patients, understand their concerns, and develop personalized treatment plans that consider the whole person.

5. Preventive Medicine: Osteopathic medicine places significant importance on preventive care to maintain health and prevent illness. Osteopaths focus on promoting healthy lifestyle choices, such as proper nutrition, exercise, stress management, and sleep, to prevent disease and optimize well-being.

6. Integration of Traditional and Alternative Approaches: Osteopathic physicians are trained in both conventional medicine and osteopathic principles. They integrate evidence-based medical practices with osteopathic manipulative treatment and other alternative therapies to provide comprehensive care for their patients.

7. Collaboration with Other Healthcare Providers: Osteopaths work collaboratively with other healthcare professionals, including medical doctors, specialists, physical therapists, and mental health practitioners, to ensure patients receive the most appropriate and comprehensive care.

The holistic approach in osteopathic medicine recognizes that the mind, body, and spirit are interconnected and that addressing all aspects of a person's health is essential for optimal well-being. By combining the best of traditional medicine with osteopathic principles, osteopathic physicians strive to provide patient-centered care that addresses the root causes of illness and promotes overall health and healing.

Osteopathic Manipulative Treatment (OMT)

Osteopathic Manipulative Treatment (OMT) is a hands-on therapeutic technique used by osteopathic physicians to diagnose, treat, and prevent illness or injury. OMT is a key component of osteopathic medicine and is based on the principles that the body's structure and function are interrelated and that restoring balance and mobility can promote healing and overall health.

During an OMT session, the osteopathic physician uses their hands to apply specific manual techniques to the patient's body, including muscles, joints, and soft tissues. These techniques may include stretching, gentle pressure, resistance, and manipulation. The goal of OMT is to improve the body's structural alignment, enhance blood flow, and optimize the function of the body's systems.

OMT can be used to address various conditions, including musculoskeletal problems, pain, and certain functional disorders. Some of the common conditions treated with OMT include:

1. Back pain and neck pain
2. Headaches and migraines
3. Joint pain and stiffness
4. Muscle strains and sprains
5. Postural imbalances
6. Sports injuries
7. Digestive disorders

8. Asthma and respiratory issues

The specific techniques used in OMT vary depending on the patient's condition and needs. Osteopathic physicians are trained in a wide range of manipulative techniques, and they tailor the treatment to each individual's unique case.

OMT is generally safe and well-tolerated, and it can be used as a stand-alone treatment or in conjunction with other medical interventions. It is important to note that OMT is not a replacement for conventional medical care but rather an additional tool that osteopathic physicians use to complement and enhance overall patient care.

Before performing OMT, osteopathic physicians conduct a thorough evaluation of the patient's medical history, perform physical examinations, and consider other diagnostic tests when necessary. The treatment plan is then developed based on the patient's specific needs and conditions.

It is essential to consult with a licensed and experienced osteopathic physician to determine if OMT is an appropriate treatment option for a particular condition. OMT can be a valuable tool in promoting healing, reducing pain, and improving overall well-being for many patients.

Osteopathic Interventions for Musculoskeletal Disorders

Osteopathic physicians use a variety of interventions to address musculoskeletal disorders and promote musculoskeletal health. These interventions, collectively known as Osteopathic Manipulative Treatment (OMT), are hands-on techniques that aim to restore balance and mobility in the musculoskeletal system. Here are some common OMT techniques used for musculoskeletal disorders:

1. Soft Tissue Techniques: These techniques involve gentle pressure and stretching of the muscles, ligaments, and other soft tissues to reduce muscle tension and improve tissue mobility. Examples include myofascial release and soft tissue mobilization.

2. Muscle Energy Technique (MET): MET involves active contraction of the patient's muscles against controlled resistance provided by the osteopathic physician. This technique is used to improve joint mobility and correct musculoskeletal imbalances.

3. Joint Mobilization and Manipulation: This technique involves using gentle movements or high-velocity thrusts to restore normal joint function, reduce joint stiffness, and relieve pain. Joint mobilization is a gentle technique, while joint manipulation is more forceful and usually accompanied by a popping sound.

4. Counterstrain: This technique involves placing the affected body part in a position of ease, where strain is removed from the involved tissues. This helps reduce

     pain and muscle spasm.

5. Ligamentous Articular Strain Technique (LAST): LAST involves precise stretching and manipulation of the ligaments and joint capsules to improve joint motion and reduce pain.

6. Balanced Ligamentous Tension (BLT): BLT is used to release tension in ligaments and joint capsules by applying gentle forces in specific directions.

7. High-Velocity Low-Amplitude (HVLA) Thrust: HVLA thrust is a quick, controlled thrusting movement applied to specific joints to restore joint motion and alleviate restrictions.

Osteopathic interventions for musculoskeletal disorders are generally safe and effective when performed by trained and licensed osteopathic physicians. OMT can be used to treat a wide range of musculoskeletal conditions, including back pain, neck pain, joint pain, sports injuries, and more. It is essential to have a thorough evaluation by an osteopathic physician to determine the most appropriate OMT techniques for a specific condition. OMT is often used in combination with other treatment modalities to provide comprehensive care and promote overall musculoskeletal health.

Emergency Medicine

Emergency medicine is a medical specialty that focuses on the diagnosis and treatment of acute illnesses and injuries that require immediate medical attention. Emergency medicine physicians, also known as emergency room (ER) doctors, work in hospital emergency departments, providing rapid assessment and care to patients in critical condition.

Key aspects of emergency medicine include:

1. Trauma Care: Emergency medicine physicians are trained to manage and stabilize patients with traumatic injuries, such as car accidents, falls, or gunshot wounds. They work alongside other healthcare professionals to provide life-saving interventions in emergency situations.

2. Critical Care: Emergency medicine physicians are skilled in managing critically ill patients who require intensive medical care, such as those experiencing heart attacks, strokes, or respiratory distress.

3. Rapid Evaluation: In the emergency department, time is critical. Emergency medicine physicians are trained to quickly assess patients and identify the most urgent medical needs.

4. Diagnostic Skills: Emergency medicine physicians must be proficient in making quick and accurate diagnoses based on limited information, often using laboratory tests, imaging, and physical examinations.

5. Treatment and Procedures: Emergency medicine physicians are trained to perform a wide range of medical procedures, such as suturing wounds, starting

intravenous (IV) lines, and inserting breathing tubes.

6. Triage: In busy emergency departments, patients are triaged based on the severity of their condition. Emergency medicine physicians help prioritize patient care based on the level of urgency.

7. Disaster Preparedness: Emergency medicine physicians play a crucial role in disaster response and management, ensuring that healthcare resources are allocated efficiently during emergencies and mass casualty incidents.

8. Teamwork: Emergency medicine physicians work closely with other healthcare professionals, including nurses, paramedics, radiologists, and surgeons, to provide comprehensive care to patients.

Emergency medicine is a high-pressure and fast-paced specialty that requires excellent communication, decision-making, and problem-solving skills. The goal of emergency medicine is to provide timely and effective care to patients in critical situations and stabilize them for further treatment or admission to the hospital if needed.

Acute Care and Emergency Interventions

Acute care and emergency interventions in the context of medicine refer to the immediate and urgent treatment provided to patients who are experiencing sudden and severe medical conditions or injuries. These interventions are designed to stabilize the patient's condition and prevent further harm until more definitive care can be provided.

Key components of acute care and emergency interventions include:

1. Rapid Assessment: Healthcare providers quickly assess the patient's vital signs, symptoms, and medical history to identify the underlying cause of the acute condition.
2. Life Support: In critical situations, life-saving interventions such as cardiopulmonary resuscitation (CPR) and advanced cardiac life support (ACLS) may be necessary to maintain vital functions.
3. Monitoring: Continuous monitoring of the patient's vital signs, such as heart rate, blood pressure, and oxygen levels, helps healthcare providers track the patient's response to treatment and identify any changes in their condition.
4. Diagnostic Testing: Laboratory tests, imaging studies (e.g., X-rays, CT scans), and other diagnostic procedures are often performed to aid in the diagnosis and guide treatment decisions.
5. Medication Administration: Emergency medications may be administered to manage pain, control severe symptoms, or address life-threatening conditions.

6. Procedures: Various medical procedures may be performed in emergency situations, such as wound care, intubation, and chest tube insertion.
7. Triage: Patients are triaged based on the severity of their condition, ensuring that those with the most critical needs receive immediate attention.
8. Timely Communication: Effective communication among healthcare team members is vital to coordinate care and ensure prompt treatment.
9. Continuity of Care: After stabilization, patients may be transferred to the appropriate department or facility for ongoing care and management of their condition.

Acute care and emergency interventions are typically provided in emergency departments, intensive care units (ICUs), and other critical care settings. Healthcare professionals, including emergency medicine physicians, critical care nurses, and other specialists, work collaboratively to deliver timely and high-quality care to patients in acute situations.

The main goal of acute care and emergency interventions is to stabilize the patient's condition, prevent complications, and initiate appropriate treatments to improve outcomes. Once the acute phase is managed, patients may require further medical management, rehabilitation, or long-term care as needed.

Triage and Trauma Management

Triage and trauma management are critical components of emergency medicine and are essential in providing timely and appropriate care to patients with acute and life-threatening injuries or conditions. These processes help healthcare providers prioritize patients based on the severity of their condition and allocate resources efficiently to save lives and optimize outcomes.

Triage: Triage is the systematic process of sorting patients based on the severity of their injuries or illnesses to determine the order in which they should receive medical care. During a mass casualty incident or a large-scale emergency, triage helps ensure that limited resources are used effectively to treat the most critically ill or injured patients first. Triage categories often used are:

1. Immediate (Red): Patients with life-threatening injuries or conditions that require immediate intervention to save their lives.
2. Delayed (Yellow): Patients with significant injuries or conditions that are not immediately life-threatening but require medical attention.
3. Minimal (Green): Patients with minor injuries or illnesses who can wait for treatment without their conditions worsening.
4. Expectant (Black): Patients with injuries or illnesses that are so severe that survival is unlikely even with medical intervention. In some cases, this category may also include those who are deceased.

Trauma Management: Trauma management involves providing immediate medical care to patients with severe injuries resulting from accidents, falls, or other traumatic events. It typically follows the Advanced Trauma Life Support (ATLS) principles and includes the following steps:

1. Primary Survey: A rapid assessment of the patient's airway, breathing, circulation, disability (neurological status), and exposure to identify life-threatening injuries and intervene immediately if needed.
2. Airway Management: Ensuring a patent airway and providing assisted ventilation or intubation if necessary.
3. Breathing Support: Providing supplemental oxygen and addressing any breathing difficulties, such as chest injuries or tension pneumothorax.
4. Circulatory Support: Managing shock, controlling bleeding, and administering intravenous fluids and medications as needed.
5. Disability Evaluation: Assessing the patient's neurological status and identifying any signs of head or spinal cord injury.
6. Exposure/Environmental Control: Keeping the patient warm and protecting against further injury or environmental factors.
7. Secondary Survey: A more detailed assessment to identify additional injuries or conditions that may not have been apparent during the primary survey.
8. Imaging and Diagnostic Studies: Obtaining X-rays, CT scans, or other diagnostic tests to further evaluate injuries.
9. Definitive Care: Initiating appropriate treatments or surgical interventions based on the identified injuries.

Triage and trauma management are challenging tasks that require quick decision-making, effective communication, and teamwork among healthcare providers. By efficiently identifying and treating the most critical cases first, these processes save lives and improve outcomes for patients in emergency situations.

Critical Decision Making in Emergency Situations

Critical decision-making in emergency situations is a crucial skill that healthcare providers must possess to provide prompt and effective care to patients facing life-threatening conditions. These situations often involve high stakes, time constraints, and rapidly changing circumstances, making the decision-making process even more challenging. Here are some key principles of critical decision-making in emergency situations:

1. Rapid Assessment: Conduct a quick but thorough assessment of the patient's condition, focusing on identifying life-threatening issues. Use standardized protocols like the ABCDE approach (Airway, Breathing, Circulation, Disability, Exposure) to prioritize interventions.

2. Gather Information: Gather as much relevant information as possible from the patient, bystanders, and medical history. Use vital signs, physical examination findings, and diagnostic tests to make informed decisions.

3. Prioritization: Prioritize actions based on the severity of the patient's condition. Address life-threatening issues first before moving on to less urgent concerns.

4. Utilize Teamwork: Effective communication and collaboration are essential in emergency situations. Work closely with other healthcare team members to coordinate efforts and pool resources.

5. Risk-Benefit Analysis: Weigh the potential risks and

benefits of each intervention. Consider the potential consequences of actions and the potential harm caused by inaction.

6. Adaptability: Emergency situations can change rapidly. Be flexible and willing to adjust the treatment plan based on the patient's response and evolving circumstances.

7. Stay Calm and Composed: Maintain a composed and focused demeanor during high-stress situations. Panic can impair decision-making and hinder patient care.

8. Ethical Considerations: Be aware of ethical principles, such as beneficence (doing good) and non-maleficence (doing no harm), when making decisions.

9. Use Evidence-Based Guidelines: Rely on evidence-based guidelines and best practices to guide decision-making whenever possible.

10. Communicate Clearly: Communicate your decisions clearly and concisely to the healthcare team and patients or their families, ensuring everyone is on the same page.

11. Reflect and Learn: After the emergency situation, take the time to debrief and reflect on the decisions made. Identify areas for improvement and learn from the experience to enhance future performance.

12. Practice and Training: Regularly participate in emergency simulation training and continuous education to sharpen critical decision-making skills.

In emergency situations, healthcare providers must be able to quickly analyze the situation, prioritize actions, and make sound decisions. The ability to stay focused, communicate effectively, and draw upon one's knowledge and experience are essential for successful outcomes in critical situations.

Family Practice

Family practice is a medical specialty that focuses on providing comprehensive and continuous healthcare to individuals and families across all ages and genders. Family practitioners, also known as family physicians or general practitioners, are primary care providers who play a central role in the healthcare system.

Key aspects of family practice include:

1. Scope of Care: Family practitioners are trained to address a wide range of health issues and provide preventive, diagnostic, and therapeutic services for acute and chronic conditions. They can treat patients of all ages, from newborns to elderly individuals.

2. Continuity of Care: Family practitioners emphasize long-term relationships with their patients, offering continuous care over time. This approach allows them to better understand patients' medical history, lifestyle, and unique healthcare needs.

3. Preventive Medicine: Preventive care is a cornerstone of family practice. Family practitioners focus on promoting healthy lifestyles, disease prevention, and early detection through routine screenings and vaccinations.

4. Health Maintenance: Family practitioners provide routine health check-ups and wellness visits to monitor patients' health status and address any emerging health concerns promptly.

5. Management of Chronic Conditions: Family practitioners manage chronic diseases, such

as diabetes, hypertension, asthma, and heart disease, through ongoing monitoring, medication management, and lifestyle modifications.

6. Referrals and Coordination: When specialized care is required, family practitioners coordinate with other healthcare specialists and ensure seamless transitions for their patients.

7. Patient-Centered Approach: Family practitioners adopt a patient-centered approach, involving patients in their healthcare decisions and considering their preferences, values, and beliefs.

8. Holistic Care: Family practitioners consider the physical, emotional, and social aspects of patients' health to provide comprehensive and holistic care.

9. Health Education: Family practitioners educate patients and their families about healthy behaviors, disease management, and self-care practices to empower them to take charge of their health.

10. Community Medicine: Family practitioners often have a strong connection to the communities they serve, promoting health awareness and engaging in community health initiatives.

Family practice is a versatile specialty that plays a critical role in promoting health, preventing illness, and managing a wide array of medical conditions. By providing comprehensive and patient-centered care, family practitioners contribute to the overall well-being of individuals and families throughout their lives.

Comprehensive Primary Care and Preventive Services

Comprehensive primary care and preventive services are fundamental components of healthcare that focus on promoting and maintaining the overall health and well-being of individuals. These services are typically provided by primary care providers, such as family physicians, internists, pediatricians, and nurse practitioners. They play a crucial role in preventing, identifying, and managing health conditions, as well as addressing the physical, emotional, and social needs of patients.

Key aspects of comprehensive primary care and preventive services include:

1. Preventive Care: Primary care providers offer a range of preventive services, including immunizations, screenings for various conditions (e.g., cancer, hypertension, diabetes), and counseling on lifestyle modifications (e.g., diet, exercise, smoking cessation).
2. Health Promotion: Primary care providers focus on promoting healthy behaviors and lifestyle choices to prevent the onset of chronic diseases and improve overall health outcomes.
3. Early Detection and Diagnosis: Regular check-ups and health assessments help identify potential health issues early, allowing for timely intervention and management.
4. Continuity of Care: Primary care providers establish

long-term relationships with their patients, ensuring ongoing care and support. Continuity of care allows providers to better understand patients' medical history and individual needs.

5. Holistic Approach: Comprehensive primary care takes into account not only the physical health of patients but also their emotional, mental, and social well-being. It addresses the whole person and their unique healthcare needs.

6. Chronic Disease Management: Primary care providers are instrumental in managing chronic diseases, such as diabetes, hypertension, asthma, and obesity, through ongoing monitoring and treatment.

7. Patient Education: Patients receive guidance and education about their health conditions, medications, and lifestyle modifications to actively participate in their healthcare decision-making.

8. Coordination of Care: Primary care providers coordinate care with specialists and other healthcare professionals to ensure that patients receive appropriate and timely treatment for complex conditions.

9. Well-Child Visits: Pediatric primary care focuses on monitoring the growth and development of children through regular well-child visits and providing immunizations.

10. Addressing Mental Health: Primary care providers screen for mental health conditions and provide counseling or referral to mental health specialists when needed.

Comprehensive primary care and preventive services are essential in promoting health and reducing healthcare costs by preventing or detecting health issues early, leading to better health outcomes and improved quality of life. These services emphasize the importance of proactive and patient-centered care, fostering a positive and collaborative patient-provider relationship.

Managing Chronic Diseases in Family Practice

Managing chronic diseases in family practice is a critical aspect of primary care, as chronic conditions are prevalent and require ongoing care and monitoring. Some common chronic diseases managed in family practice include diabetes, hypertension, asthma, chronic obstructive pulmonary disease (COPD), heart disease, and arthritis, among others. The goal of managing chronic diseases is to improve patients' quality of life, prevent complications, and optimize their overall health outcomes.

Here are some key approaches to managing chronic diseases in family practice:

1. Comprehensive Assessment: Primary care providers conduct a thorough assessment of the patient's medical history, family history, lifestyle, and current health status to understand the extent of the chronic condition and its impact on the patient's life.
2. Goal Setting: Establishing clear and achievable health goals with the patient is essential. These goals may include controlling blood pressure, maintaining blood glucose levels within the target range, improving lung function, or reducing pain and inflammation.
3. Medication Management: Prescribing and managing medications is a vital aspect of chronic disease management. Family physicians ensure that patients are on appropriate medications, monitor their response, and adjust dosages as needed.

4. Lifestyle Modifications: Encouraging and supporting patients to adopt healthy lifestyle habits can significantly impact chronic disease management. This includes promoting regular exercise, a balanced diet, smoking cessation, and stress management.

5. Self-Management Education: Providing patients with the necessary knowledge and skills to manage their chronic conditions effectively is crucial. Education may include self-monitoring techniques, medication administration, recognizing symptoms of exacerbation, and knowing when to seek medical help.

6. Regular Follow-up: Scheduling regular follow-up visits allows family physicians to monitor the patient's progress, assess the effectiveness of treatment plans, and make adjustments as needed.

7. Patient Engagement: Engaging patients in their care decision-making process empowers them to take an active role in managing their health. Family physicians listen to their patients' concerns, address their questions, and involve them in developing individualized care plans.

8. Care Coordination: Chronic disease management often involves coordination with other healthcare professionals, such as specialists, nurses, dietitians, and pharmacists, to ensure a comprehensive approach to patient care.

9. Use of Technology: Utilizing electronic health records (EHRs) and digital health tools can improve communication and information sharing between patients and healthcare providers. It also aids in tracking patients' progress and treatment outcomes.

10. Patient Support Groups: Encouraging patients to participate in support groups for their specific chronic conditions can provide additional emotional support and resources for coping with the challenges of living with chronic diseases.

By implementing a patient-centered and multidisciplinary approach, family practitioners can effectively manage chronic diseases, improve patients' quality of life, and reduce the burden of chronic conditions on the healthcare system.

The Role of Family Practitioners in Healthcare Systems

Family practitioners, also known as family physicians or general practitioners, play a crucial role in healthcare systems worldwide. They serve as primary care providers who offer comprehensive medical care to patients of all ages and genders. The role of family practitioners encompasses various aspects that contribute to the overall well-being of patients and the efficiency of healthcare systems:

1. First Point of Contact: Family practitioners are often the first healthcare professionals that patients visit when they have health concerns. They provide initial evaluations, diagnose conditions, and initiate appropriate treatment plans. As primary care providers, they are essential for early detection and prevention of diseases.

2. Continuity of Care: Family practitioners are focused on building long-term relationships with their patients. This continuity of care allows them to develop a deep understanding of their patients' medical history, family dynamics, and individual health needs, leading to personalized and effective healthcare.

3. Preventive Medicine: Family practitioners emphasize preventive medicine and health promotion. They educate patients about healthy lifestyle choices, disease prevention, and the importance of regular check-ups and screenings to identify health risks early on.

4. Diagnosis and Treatment: Family practitioners are skilled in diagnosing a wide range of medical conditions. They provide appropriate treatment, manage chronic diseases, and refer patients to specialists when necessary for more specialized care.

5. Holistic Approach: Family practitioners take a holistic approach to patient care, considering not only the physical health but also the emotional, social, and psychological well-being of their patients. This comprehensive approach contributes to better overall health outcomes.

6. Care Coordination: Family practitioners serve as the central point of contact for their patients' healthcare needs. They coordinate care across different specialties and healthcare settings, ensuring that patients receive integrated and cohesive care.

7. Health Promotion and Patient Education: Family practitioners educate patients about healthy habits, disease management, and medication adherence. They empower patients to make informed decisions about their health and actively participate in their care.

8. Managing Chronic Conditions: Family practitioners are skilled in managing chronic conditions such as diabetes, hypertension, asthma, and heart disease. They work closely with patients to develop individualized care plans to optimize health outcomes.

9. Advocacy and Public Health: Family practitioners often play an advocacy role in public health initiatives and disease prevention programs. They contribute to the development of health policies, promote vaccination campaigns, and advocate for health equity.

10. Cost-Effective Care: Family practitioners provide cost-effective healthcare by addressing most of their patients' health needs at the primary care level. This reduces unnecessary visits to specialists and

hospitalizations, leading to overall cost savings for the healthcare system.

In summary, family practitioners are vital components of healthcare systems, serving as the cornerstone of primary care. Their comprehensive and patient-centered approach, emphasis on preventive medicine, and ability to manage a wide range of health conditions contribute to improving patient outcomes and promoting the overall health of communities.

Occupational & Industrial Medicine

Occupational and Industrial Medicine, also known as Occupational Medicine, is a medical specialty focused on the health and well-being of workers in various occupational settings. It deals with the prevention, diagnosis, and treatment of work-related injuries and illnesses, as well as the promotion of overall health and safety in the workplace. Occupational medicine practitioners work to protect both the health of individual workers and the productivity of the workforce as a whole. Here are some key aspects of Occupational and Industrial Medicine:

1. Occupational Health Services: Occupational medicine professionals provide a wide range of health services to workers, including pre-employment medical evaluations, periodic health assessments, and medical surveillance to monitor the health of employees exposed to certain occupational hazards.

2. Workplace Injury Management: They manage work-related injuries, including musculoskeletal disorders, cuts, burns, and other accidents that occur on the job. They help injured workers recover and safely return to work.

3. Occupational Hazards: Occupational medicine specialists identify and assess workplace hazards, such as exposure to chemicals, noise, radiation, and repetitive motions, that can adversely affect workers' health. They work with employers to develop strategies for minimizing these risks.

4. Ergonomics and Workplace Design: Occupational

medicine professionals evaluate workplace ergonomics and design to ensure that the work environment is optimized for worker comfort, safety, and efficiency.

5. Occupational Health Promotion: They promote health and wellness among workers, emphasizing the importance of healthy lifestyle choices, stress management, and disease prevention.

6. Fitness for Duty Evaluations: Occupational medicine practitioners assess whether workers are physically and mentally fit to perform specific job duties, particularly in safety-sensitive roles.

7. Disability Management: They collaborate with employers, insurers, and rehabilitation specialists to manage disability cases and facilitate the return-to-work process for employees with work-related injuries or illnesses.

8. Occupational Toxicology: Occupational medicine specialists assess and manage exposure to hazardous substances and chemicals in the workplace, ensuring proper protection and safety measures are in place.

9. Worksite Health Programs: They develop and implement health and wellness programs tailored to the specific needs of the workforce, aiming to improve overall health and productivity.

10. Regulatory Compliance: Occupational medicine professionals ensure that employers comply with relevant occupational health and safety regulations to maintain a safe working environment for employees.

Occupational and Industrial Medicine plays a vital role in promoting a healthy and safe work environment, reducing workplace injuries and illnesses, and enhancing the overall well-being of the workforce. By focusing on prevention and early intervention, occupational medicine specialists contribute to reducing healthcare costs and improving the productivity of organizations.

Occupational Health and Workplace Safety

Occupational health and workplace safety are crucial aspects of ensuring the well-being of employees and creating a safe and productive work environment. Here are key components of occupational health and workplace safety:

1. Risk Assessment: Employers conduct risk assessments to identify potential hazards in the workplace that could harm employees' health or safety. This includes evaluating physical, chemical, biological, ergonomic, and psychosocial factors.

2. Safety Training: Employers provide regular safety training to employees to raise awareness of potential hazards and educate them on safe work practices and emergency procedures.

3. Personal Protective Equipment (PPE): Employers ensure that appropriate personal protective equipment, such as safety helmets, gloves, goggles, and masks, is provided to employees to protect them from potential hazards.

4. Health Surveillance: Occupational health professionals conduct health surveillance to monitor the health of employees who may be exposed to certain workplace hazards, such as noise, chemicals, or radiation.

5. Ergonomics: Employers consider ergonomic principles in the design of workstations and equipment to reduce physical strain and prevent musculoskeletal disorders.

6. Hazard Communication: Employers implement clear communication systems to inform employees about the potential hazards in the workplace and the measures taken to control them.

7. Emergency Response Planning: Employers develop and communicate emergency response plans to employees to ensure a swift and coordinated response in case of accidents or emergencies.

8. Worksite Inspections: Regular worksite inspections help identify safety issues and ensure that safety measures are implemented and followed.

9. Health and Wellness Programs: Employers may offer health and wellness programs to promote employee well-being and prevent chronic health conditions.

10. Incident Reporting and Investigation: Employers establish a process for employees to report incidents and near misses, followed by thorough investigations to identify the root causes and prevent future occurrences.

11. Compliance with Regulations: Employers must comply with local, national, and international occupational health and safety regulations to maintain a safe working environment.

12. Workplace Culture: Fostering a safety-conscious workplace culture where employees feel comfortable reporting safety concerns and participating in safety initiatives is crucial.

By prioritizing occupational health and workplace safety, employers can protect their employees from harm, reduce the risk of accidents and injuries, enhance productivity, and create a positive work environment. Additionally, adherence to safety standards can result in reduced absenteeism, lower healthcare costs, and increased employee morale and satisfaction.

Occupational Medicine Interventions and Injury Management

Occupational medicine focuses on the prevention and management of work-related injuries and illnesses. Here are some key interventions and injury management strategies used in occupational medicine:

1. Pre-employment Medical Examinations: Before hiring new employees, employers may conduct pre-employment medical examinations to ensure that individuals are fit to perform the job requirements safely.

2. Health and Safety Training: Providing employees with comprehensive health and safety training helps them understand potential workplace hazards and how to avoid injuries.

3. Workplace Ergonomics: Occupational medicine professionals assess the ergonomics of workstations and job tasks to optimize the work environment and reduce the risk of musculoskeletal injuries.

4. Injury Prevention Programs: Developing injury prevention programs specific to the workplace can reduce the incidence of work-related injuries. These programs may include safe work practices, proper lifting techniques, and equipment use.

5. Health Promotion and Wellness: Implementing health promotion and wellness programs can improve employees' overall health and well-being, reducing the risk of chronic conditions and injuries.

6. Return-to-Work Programs: After an employee experiences a work-related injury or illness, occupational medicine professionals may design return-to-work programs to facilitate a safe and gradual return to full work duties.

7. Case Management: Occupational medicine specialists may be involved in case management, coordinating medical care and facilitating communication among healthcare providers, employers, and insurers to ensure optimal treatment and recovery for injured workers.

8. Worksite Health Clinics: Some companies establish onsite health clinics staffed with occupational medicine professionals to provide immediate care for workplace injuries and illnesses.

9. Injury Reporting and Investigation: Employers maintain a system for reporting and investigating workplace injuries to identify the root causes and implement corrective actions.

10. Rehabilitation Services: Occupational medicine practitioners may provide rehabilitation services to injured workers, including physical therapy and occupational therapy, to aid in their recovery and restore function.

11. Worksite Assessments: Regular worksite assessments help identify potential hazards and areas for improvement in workplace safety.

12. Collaborating with Employers: Occupational medicine professionals work closely with employers to develop and implement safety policies and programs, fostering a culture of safety in the workplace.

13. Utilizing Technology: Implementing technology in injury management, such as electronic health records and telemedicine, can improve communication and streamline care.

Occupational medicine plays a critical role in safeguarding the health and well-being of employees and promoting a safe work environment. By proactively addressing workplace hazards and promptly managing injuries, occupational medicine interventions can reduce the risk of work-related health issues and contribute to a healthier and more productive workforce.

Industrial Hygiene and Occupational Health Assessments

Industrial hygiene is a branch of occupational health and safety that focuses on identifying and controlling workplace hazards to protect workers' health. Occupational health assessments, often conducted by industrial hygienists, involve evaluating workplace conditions and employee exposures to potential health risks. Here are key components of industrial hygiene and occupational health assessments:

1. Hazard Identification: Industrial hygienists identify potential hazards in the workplace, including chemical, biological, physical, and ergonomic hazards. This may involve inspecting work areas, reviewing safety data sheets, and interviewing workers.

2. Exposure Assessment: Industrial hygienists measure and evaluate employee exposures to hazardous substances and conditions. They use various sampling techniques to monitor airborne contaminants, noise levels, vibration, and other physical stressors.

3. Risk Assessment: After collecting exposure data, industrial hygienists assess the risks associated with specific workplace hazards. They compare the exposure levels to occupational exposure limits and health-based guidelines.

4. Control Measures: Based on the assessment results, industrial hygienists recommend control measures to minimize or eliminate exposure to hazards. This may involve engineering controls, administrative controls,

and personal protective equipment (PPE).

5. Health Surveillance: Occupational health assessments include monitoring workers' health to detect early signs of work-related illnesses or diseases. This may involve periodic medical examinations and health screenings.

6. Ergonomic Assessments: Industrial hygienists conduct ergonomic assessments to evaluate the physical demands of job tasks and identify potential risks of musculoskeletal disorders. They may suggest workplace modifications to improve ergonomics.

7. Training and Education: Industrial hygienists provide training and educational programs for workers, supervisors, and management to increase awareness of workplace hazards and safe work practices.

8. Compliance with Regulations: Industrial hygienists ensure that the workplace complies with relevant health and safety regulations and standards.

9. Hazard Communication: They assist in developing and implementing hazard communication programs to inform workers about the hazards present in the workplace.

10. Emergency Preparedness: Industrial hygienists participate in developing emergency response plans and procedures to address potential hazardous incidents.

11. Data Analysis and Reporting: They analyze assessment data and prepare comprehensive reports outlining the findings, recommendations, and action plans.

12. Continuous Monitoring: Industrial hygienists may conduct regular follow-up assessments to evaluate the effectiveness of control measures and ensure ongoing compliance with health and safety standards.

By conducting industrial hygiene and occupational health assessments, organizations can proactively identify and mitigate workplace hazards, protect the health and safety of their employees, and maintain a productive and sustainable workforce.

Physical Medicine & Rehabilitation

Physical Medicine and Rehabilitation (PM&R), also known as physiatry, is a medical specialty focused on restoring and enhancing the functional abilities of individuals who have physical impairments or disabilities resulting from injuries, illnesses, or chronic medical conditions. PM&R physicians, known as physiatrists, utilize a comprehensive and patient-centered approach to improve the quality of life and functional independence of their patients. Here are key aspects of Physical Medicine and Rehabilitation:

1. Assessment and Diagnosis: Physiatrists evaluate patients through comprehensive assessments, including medical history reviews, physical examinations, and functional evaluations. They diagnose the underlying cause of the functional impairment and develop personalized treatment plans.

2. Multidisciplinary Care: PM&R emphasizes a team-based approach to care, collaborating with various healthcare professionals, such as physical therapists, occupational therapists, speech therapists, psychologists, and social workers, to provide comprehensive and integrated care.

3. Treatment Modalities: Physiatrists use a wide range of treatment modalities, including physical therapy, occupational therapy, speech therapy, medications, assistive devices, orthotics, and prosthetics. They may also employ interventional procedures, such as joint injections or nerve blocks, to manage pain and

improve function.

4. Pain Management: Physiatrists specialize in managing acute and chronic pain related to musculoskeletal conditions, neurological disorders, and other medical conditions. They utilize various techniques to alleviate pain, enhance function, and improve the overall quality of life.

5. Neurorehabilitation: PM&R focuses on the rehabilitation of individuals with neurological conditions, such as stroke, spinal cord injuries, traumatic brain injuries, multiple sclerosis, and cerebral palsy. Neurorehabilitation aims to maximize recovery and help patients regain lost abilities.

6. Orthopedic Rehabilitation: Physiatrists address orthopedic conditions, such as fractures, musculoskeletal injuries, and joint replacements. They work with patients to optimize healing, restore mobility, and improve function.

7. Sports Medicine: Physiatrists play a vital role in the sports medicine field, providing non-surgical care for sports-related injuries and optimizing athletes' performance and recovery.

8. Geriatric Rehabilitation: PM&R also caters to the needs of older adults, focusing on preserving independence, enhancing mobility, and addressing age-related functional decline.

9. Amputee Rehabilitation: Physiatrists work with amputees to provide comprehensive care, including fitting and training with prosthetic devices to maximize functionality and mobility.

10. Spinal Cord Injury Rehabilitation: Physiatrists specialize in the management and rehabilitation of patients with spinal cord injuries, helping them adapt to their new circumstances and improve their quality of life.

11. Patient Education: PM&R physicians

educate patients and their families about their conditions, treatment options, and self-management strategies to promote active participation in the rehabilitation process.

12.   Vocational Rehabilitation: Physiatrists assist patients in transitioning back to work or finding suitable employment opportunities following an injury or illness.

Physical Medicine and Rehabilitation focuses on enhancing patients' physical, emotional, and social well-being by maximizing their functional abilities and improving their overall quality of life. The specialty plays a crucial role in the comprehensive care of individuals with disabilities and physical impairments across the lifespan.

Rehabilitation Medicine and Functional Restoration

Rehabilitation Medicine, also known as Physical Medicine and Rehabilitation (PM&R), is a medical specialty focused on restoring and optimizing functional abilities and quality of life for individuals with physical impairments or disabilities. The goal of rehabilitation medicine is to help patients regain independence, mobility, and overall well-being after an injury, illness, or chronic condition. Functional restoration is a central concept within rehabilitation medicine, and it involves a comprehensive and multidisciplinary approach to patient care. Here are key aspects of Rehabilitation Medicine and functional restoration:

1. Multidisciplinary Team: Rehabilitation medicine involves a collaborative approach, bringing together a team of healthcare professionals with expertise in various areas, such as physical therapy, occupational therapy, speech therapy, social work, nursing, psychology, and other disciplines. This interdisciplinary team works together to address the diverse needs of patients.

2. Comprehensive Evaluation: Physiatrists (rehabilitation physicians) perform a thorough evaluation of patients to understand their medical history, physical impairments, functional limitations, and individual goals. This assessment helps in tailoring a personalized rehabilitation plan.

3. Individualized Treatment Plans: Based on the

evaluation, a comprehensive and individualized treatment plan is developed for each patient. The plan may include a combination of therapies, interventions, and assistive devices to address the specific functional challenges and achieve optimal outcomes.

4. Physical Therapy: Physical therapy is a fundamental component of functional restoration. It involves exercises, manual therapies, and various techniques to improve strength, flexibility, balance, and mobility.

5. Occupational Therapy: Occupational therapy focuses on helping patients regain skills needed for daily activities and tasks, including self-care, work, and leisure. It aims to enhance independence and quality of life.

6. Speech Therapy: Speech therapy addresses communication and swallowing difficulties, which may arise due to neurological conditions, injuries, or surgeries.

7. Pain Management: Rehabilitation medicine specialists are trained in managing acute and chronic pain related to various conditions. Pain management techniques may include medications, interventional procedures, and non-pharmacological approaches.

8. Assistive Devices and Technology: Rehabilitation professionals may prescribe and teach the use of assistive devices, such as wheelchairs, prosthetics, orthotics, and adaptive tools, to promote independence and function.

9. Neurological Rehabilitation: Functional restoration is particularly important for patients with neurological conditions, such as stroke, traumatic brain injury, spinal cord injury, multiple sclerosis, and Parkinson's disease. Neurorehabilitation aims to promote neuroplasticity and improve function in affected areas.

10.   Psychological Support: Rehabilitation medicine recognizes the emotional and psychological aspects of recovery. Psychological support and counseling are provided to patients and their families to cope with the challenges of rehabilitation.

11.   Progressive Goal Setting: Functional restoration involves setting realistic and progressive goals for patients. Regular reassessment and adjustment of treatment plans are made to monitor progress and achieve optimal outcomes.

12.   Long-Term Follow-Up: Rehabilitation is often an ongoing process, and long-term follow-up care is essential to ensure that patients continue to maintain and improve their functional abilities.

Functional restoration in rehabilitation medicine is an integrative and patient-centered approach that addresses physical, emotional, and social aspects of care. Through the collaborative efforts of a multidisciplinary team, patients can achieve functional independence and an improved quality of life, even in the presence of chronic conditions or disabilities.

Physical Therapy, Occupational Therapy, and Speech Therapy

Physical Therapy, Occupational Therapy, and Speech Therapy are three distinct disciplines within the field of rehabilitation medicine, each specializing in different aspects of patient care and functional restoration. Here's an overview of each:

1. Physical Therapy (PT): Physical therapy focuses on restoring and improving physical function and mobility in individuals with various musculoskeletal, neurological, and cardiopulmonary conditions. PT interventions are designed to alleviate pain, improve strength, flexibility, balance, coordination, and promote overall physical fitness. Physical therapists utilize a variety of techniques, exercises, and modalities to help patients achieve their functional goals. Common conditions treated by physical therapists include sports injuries, orthopedic conditions, stroke, spinal cord injuries, arthritis, and post-surgical rehabilitation.

2. Occupational Therapy (OT): Occupational therapy addresses the challenges that affect an individual's ability to perform daily living activities, work-related tasks, and leisure activities. Occupational therapists help patients develop the skills needed to lead independent and fulfilling lives, considering their physical, cognitive, emotional, and environmental needs. OT interventions may involve teaching adaptive techniques, recommending assistive devices,

and modifying the environment to support functional independence. Common conditions treated by occupational therapists include neurological disorders, hand injuries, developmental delays, and mental health conditions.

3. Speech Therapy (Speech-Language Pathology): Speech therapy is concerned with the assessment and treatment of communication disorders and swallowing difficulties. Speech-language pathologists (SLPs) work with individuals of all ages to improve speech articulation, language comprehension, social communication, voice quality, and fluency. Additionally, SLPs address swallowing disorders (dysphagia) to ensure safe and efficient swallowing. Speech therapy is commonly utilized for conditions such as speech delays, language disorders, stuttering, aphasia, voice disorders, and dysphagia caused by neurological conditions or other medical issues.

In many cases, patients may benefit from a combination of these therapies to address complex functional limitations and improve overall well-being. A collaborative approach among physical therapists, occupational therapists, speech-language pathologists, and other healthcare professionals often leads to more comprehensive care and better outcomes for patients. The goal of these therapies is to enhance independence, promote optimal function, and support individuals in achieving their highest level of physical, cognitive, and social abilities.

Assistive Devices and Mobility Aids

Assistive devices and mobility aids play a crucial role in enhancing the independence and quality of life for individuals with physical disabilities or mobility challenges. These devices are designed to provide support, stability, and assistance in performing daily activities and moving around safely. Here are some common types of assistive devices and mobility aids:

1. Mobility Scooters: Mobility scooters are electric-powered vehicles designed to assist individuals with mobility limitations in traveling long distances outdoors. They are particularly useful for individuals who have difficulty walking or standing for extended periods.

2. Wheelchairs: Wheelchairs are one of the most common mobility aids used by individuals with physical disabilities. They come in various types, including manual wheelchairs (propelled by the user or an attendant) and powered wheelchairs (electrically powered for independent movement).

3. Walkers: Walkers provide support and stability for individuals with balance issues or limited weight-bearing capacity. They typically consist of a metal or plastic frame with four legs and are available in different styles, including standard walkers, wheeled walkers, and rollators.

4. Canes: Canes are lightweight, single-pointed assistive devices used to improve balance and reduce the load on one leg or side of the body. They come in various styles, including straight canes, quad canes (with four

feet), and folding canes for easy transport.

5. Crutches: Crutches are often prescribed to individuals with temporary mobility challenges, such as leg injuries or post-surgery recovery. They require upper body strength and coordination to use effectively.

6. Orthoses and Prostheses: Orthoses (braces) and prostheses (artificial limbs) are custom-made devices that provide support and improve function for individuals with musculoskeletal or limb deficiencies.

7. Transfer Aids: Transfer aids, such as transfer boards and pivot discs, assist individuals with limited mobility in safely moving between different surfaces or transferring from one seated position to another.

8. Adaptive Utensils and Devices: These include specialized eating and drinking utensils designed to assist individuals with limited hand function or coordination.

9. Hearing Aids: Hearing aids are small electronic devices that improve hearing for individuals with hearing loss.

10. Visual Aids: Visual aids, including magnifiers and talking devices, support individuals with visual impairments in daily activities and reading.

11. Environmental Control Units: These devices enable individuals with physical disabilities to control various aspects of their home environment, such as lighting, temperature, and electronic devices, through voice commands or other accessible methods.

The selection of assistive devices and mobility aids is based on individual needs, functional abilities, and specific requirements. Proper assessment and fitting by healthcare professionals, such as physical therapists or occupational therapists, are essential to ensure that the chosen devices are safe, effective, and compatible with the user's lifestyle.

Reproductive Medicine & Technology

Reproductive medicine and technology encompass a wide range of medical interventions and techniques designed to assist individuals and couples in achieving successful pregnancies and addressing issues related to reproductive health. These advancements in medicine and technology have revolutionized the field of fertility treatment and reproductive care. Here are some key aspects of reproductive medicine and technology:

1. In Vitro Fertilization (IVF): IVF is one of the most well-known and widely used assisted reproductive technologies. It involves fertilizing eggs with sperm outside the body in a laboratory setting and transferring the resulting embryos into the uterus for implantation. IVF is often recommended for couples with infertility issues, such as blocked fallopian tubes, low sperm count, or unexplained infertility.

2. Intracytoplasmic Sperm Injection (ICSI): ICSI is a specialized form of IVF that involves injecting a single sperm directly into an egg to facilitate fertilization. It is commonly used in cases of male infertility or when traditional IVF methods have not resulted in successful fertilization.

3. Assisted Hatching: Assisted hatching is a technique used during IVF in which a small hole is made in the outer shell (zona pellucida) of the embryo to facilitate its implantation in the uterus.

4. Preimplantation Genetic Testing (PGT): PGT is a process that allows the screening of embryos for genetic abnormalities before they are transferred to

the uterus. It can help identify embryos with a higher chance of successful implantation and reduce the risk of passing on genetic disorders to offspring.

5. Egg Freezing and Fertility Preservation: Egg freezing allows women to preserve their fertility by freezing and storing their eggs for later use. This can be beneficial for women who want to delay childbearing due to personal or medical reasons.

6. Sperm and Embryo Cryopreservation: Sperm and embryo cryopreservation involve freezing and storing sperm or embryos for future use in fertility treatments.

7. Gamete and Embryo Donation: In cases of severe male or female infertility, couples may consider using donated eggs, sperm, or embryos from third-party donors to achieve pregnancy.

8. Surrogacy: Surrogacy is an arrangement in which a woman (the surrogate) carries and gives birth to a child on behalf of another individual or couple. This can be an option for individuals or couples who are unable to carry a pregnancy themselves.

9. Reproductive Endocrinology: Reproductive endocrinology is a specialized field within reproductive medicine that focuses on the hormonal aspects of reproductive health and fertility.

10. Minimally Invasive Reproductive Surgery: Minimally invasive surgical techniques, such as laparoscopy and hysteroscopy, can be used to diagnose and treat certain reproductive conditions, such as endometriosis, uterine fibroids, and tubal blockages.

11. Genetic Counseling: Genetic counseling is an essential component of reproductive medicine that involves providing individuals and couples with information about the genetic risks and implications of certain reproductive choices.

Reproductive medicine and technology have opened up new possibilities for individuals and couples facing challenges in conceiving a child. These advancements continue to evolve, offering hope and solutions for those seeking to build their families. However, it is essential to approach reproductive medicine with careful consideration, guided by qualified healthcare professionals, to ensure the best possible outcomes and ethical practices.

Assisted Reproductive Technologies (ART)

Assisted Reproductive Technologies (ART) are medical procedures and techniques designed to assist individuals and couples in achieving pregnancy when natural conception is not possible or has not been successful. These advanced reproductive treatments have revolutionized the field of fertility and have helped many individuals and couples realize their dreams of having children. Some common ART procedures include:

1. In Vitro Fertilization (IVF): IVF is the most well-known and widely used ART procedure. It involves the retrieval of eggs from the woman's ovaries, fertilization of the eggs with sperm in a laboratory, and the transfer of resulting embryos back into the woman's uterus for implantation.

2. Intracytoplasmic Sperm Injection (ICSI): ICSI is a specialized form of IVF that involves injecting a single sperm directly into an egg to facilitate fertilization. It is often used in cases of male infertility or when traditional IVF methods have not resulted in successful fertilization.

3. Intrauterine Insemination (IUI): IUI is a procedure in which specially prepared sperm is placed directly into the woman's uterus during her fertile period to improve the chances of fertilization.

4. Preimplantation Genetic Testing (PGT): PGT is a technique used during IVF to screen embryos for

genetic abnormalities before implantation. It can help identify healthy embryos and reduce the risk of passing on genetic disorders to offspring.

5. Egg Freezing: Egg freezing, also known as oocyte cryopreservation, allows women to preserve their fertility by freezing and storing their eggs for future use. This is often chosen by women who want to delay childbearing for personal or medical reasons.

6. Sperm Cryopreservation: Sperm cryopreservation involves freezing and storing sperm for future use, which is particularly beneficial for men who are facing treatments that may affect their fertility or for those who want to preserve their sperm before undergoing a vasectomy.

7. Embryo Cryopreservation: Embryo cryopreservation is the freezing and storing of excess embryos from IVF procedures for future use. This allows individuals or couples to have additional attempts at pregnancy without going through a complete IVF cycle.

8. Gamete and Embryo Donation: ART allows the use of donated eggs, sperm, or embryos from third-party donors to achieve pregnancy for individuals or couples with infertility issues.

9. Surrogacy: Surrogacy involves a woman (the surrogate) carrying and giving birth to a child on behalf of another individual or couple. It can be an option for those who are unable to carry a pregnancy themselves.

Assisted Reproductive Technologies have significantly increased the chances of achieving pregnancy and parenthood for many individuals and couples. However, it is crucial to seek guidance from qualified fertility specialists and reproductive health professionals to understand the most suitable ART options and ensure ethical and safe practices throughout the process.

In Vitro Fertilization (IVF) and Fertility Preservation

In Vitro Fertilization (IVF) is a form of assisted reproductive technology (ART) that involves the retrieval of eggs from a woman's ovaries, fertilization of the eggs with sperm in a laboratory dish, and the transfer of resulting embryos back into the woman's uterus for implantation. IVF is one of the most commonly used and successful treatments for infertility, helping many couples and individuals achieve pregnancy.

Here is an overview of the IVF process:

1. Ovarian Stimulation: Before the IVF procedure, the woman undergoes ovarian stimulation using fertility medications to encourage the ovaries to produce multiple eggs. Monitoring and hormone level testing are conducted during this phase to track the growth and maturity of the eggs.

2. Egg Retrieval: Once the eggs reach an optimal size and maturity, a minor surgical procedure called egg retrieval is performed. A thin needle is inserted through the vaginal wall and into the ovaries to retrieve the eggs.

3. Sperm Collection: On the day of the egg retrieval, the male partner provides a semen sample. If needed, sperm can also be obtained from a sperm donor.

4. Fertilization: The retrieved eggs are combined with the sperm in a laboratory dish for fertilization. In some cases, intracytoplasmic sperm injection (ICSI) is used,

where a single sperm is directly injected into each egg.

5. Embryo Culture: After fertilization, the embryos are cultured in a laboratory for a few days to allow them to develop.
6. Embryo Transfer: The healthiest and most viable embryos are selected for transfer to the woman's uterus. This is typically done 3 to 5 days after the egg retrieval.
7. Pregnancy Test: About two weeks after the embryo transfer, a pregnancy test is conducted to determine if the procedure was successful.

Fertility Preservation: Fertility preservation is a critical aspect of reproductive medicine, especially for individuals facing potential fertility challenges due to medical treatments or personal circumstances. Fertility preservation techniques are used to preserve reproductive potential for the future.

1. Egg Freezing (Oocyte Cryopreservation): Egg freezing involves the retrieval of mature eggs from a woman's ovaries, followed by the freezing and storage of the eggs for future use. This allows women to preserve their fertility when they are not ready to conceive or are facing medical treatments that may affect their fertility.
2. Sperm Freezing (Sperm Cryopreservation): Sperm cryopreservation is the freezing and storage of sperm for future use. It is often chosen by men who are undergoing treatments that may affect their fertility or for those who want to preserve their fertility before a vasectomy.
3. Embryo Freezing (Embryo Cryopreservation): Excess embryos created during an IVF cycle can be cryopreserved and stored for future use, allowing individuals or couples to attempt pregnancy again without undergoing a full IVF cycle.

4. Ovarian Tissue Freezing: In some cases, ovarian tissue can be removed and frozen for future transplantation or reimplantation after medical treatments.

Fertility preservation techniques have opened up new possibilities for family planning, allowing individuals to make informed decisions about their reproductive health and pursue parenthood when the time is right for them.

It is essential to consult with a qualified fertility specialist to discuss the most appropriate fertility preservation options based on individual circumstances and medical considerations.

Ethical and Legal Considerations in Reproductive Medicine

Ethical and legal considerations in reproductive medicine are crucial due to the sensitive nature of the field and the potential impact on individuals, families, and society. Here are some key ethical and legal issues in reproductive medicine:

1. Informed Consent: Patients must provide informed consent before undergoing any reproductive procedure. This includes a clear understanding of the risks, benefits, and alternatives involved in the treatment.

2. Autonomy and Decision-Making: Patients have the right to make autonomous decisions about their reproductive health, including whether to pursue assisted reproductive technologies (ART) and the disposal of embryos.

3. Embryo Disposition: Decisions regarding the disposition of unused embryos, such as donation, continued storage, or disposal, raise ethical questions about the status of embryos and their moral standing.

4. Access and Equity: Ensuring equitable access to reproductive services is an ethical concern, as these services can be expensive and may not be covered by insurance, leading to potential disparities in access to care.

5. Reproductive Rights: Reproductive rights encompass a person's right to make decisions about their reproductive health, including access to

contraception, fertility treatment, and abortion.

6. Genetic Testing and Counseling: Genetic testing is often used in reproductive medicine to screen for genetic disorders in embryos. Ethical considerations include ensuring adequate genetic counseling and informed decision-making.

7. Surrogacy and Gestational Carriers: Surrogacy arrangements involve complex ethical and legal issues related to the rights and well-being of the surrogate, intended parents, and the child.

8. Preimplantation Genetic Diagnosis (PGD): PGD involves screening embryos for genetic abnormalities before implantation. Ethical considerations include potential concerns about eugenics and the use of PGD for non-medical reasons.

9. Multifetal Pregnancy Reduction: In cases of multiple pregnancies resulting from fertility treatments, the selective reduction of embryos raises ethical and emotional dilemmas.

10. Reproductive Cloning: The ethical implications of reproductive cloning, which involves creating a genetically identical copy of a person, raise significant concerns about identity, individuality, and potential exploitation.

11. Egg and Sperm Donation: Ethical issues surround the anonymity of donors, the compensation of donors, and the rights and responsibilities of individuals conceived through donation.

12. Regulating Reproductive Medicine: Legal frameworks and regulations are essential to ensure the safety, quality, and ethical conduct of reproductive medicine practices.

13. International Surrogacy and Reproductive Tourism: Cross-border reproductive practices can lead to legal and ethical challenges due to varying laws and standards in different countries.

14.   Commercialization and Advertising: The commercialization and advertising of fertility treatments raise concerns about the potential exploitation of vulnerable individuals and the marketing of unproven interventions.

Addressing these ethical and legal issues requires ongoing dialogue, research, and consideration of the best interests of individuals and society as a whole. Ethical guidelines and legal regulations should be continually reviewed and updated to reflect advancements in science and technology while upholding the principles of autonomy, beneficence, non-maleficence, and justice in reproductive medicine.

The Expansive Landscape of Internal Medicine

Internal medicine is a broad and diverse medical specialty that encompasses the diagnosis, treatment, and management of a wide range of diseases and conditions affecting adults. The field of internal medicine includes various subspecialties and areas of focus, each dedicated to addressing specific medical issues. Here are some key areas within the expansive landscape of internal medicine:

1. General Internal Medicine: General internists provide comprehensive medical care for adults, managing a wide array of medical conditions and coordinating care for patients with multiple health concerns.
2. Cardiology: Cardiologists specialize in diagnosing and treating diseases of the heart and circulatory system, including heart attacks, heart failure, arrhythmias, and hypertension.
3. Pulmonology: Pulmonologists focus on respiratory disorders, such as asthma, chronic obstructive pulmonary disease (COPD), and interstitial lung diseases.
4. Gastroenterology: Gastroenterologists deal with disorders of the digestive system, including conditions like gastroesophageal reflux disease (GERD), inflammatory bowel disease (IBD), and liver diseases.
5. Nephrology: Nephrologists specialize in kidney diseases and conditions, such as chronic kidney disease (CKD), kidney stones, and kidney

transplantation.

6. Endocrinology: Endocrinologists diagnose and treat disorders of the endocrine system, which includes hormone-related conditions like diabetes, thyroid disorders, and hormonal imbalances.

7. Rheumatology: Rheumatologists focus on autoimmune and inflammatory disorders, including rheumatoid arthritis, lupus, and other connective tissue diseases.

8. Hematology: Hematologists specialize in disorders of the blood and blood-forming organs, such as anemia, leukemia, and clotting disorders.

9. Oncology: Medical oncologists diagnose and treat cancer, developing and coordinating cancer treatment plans that may include chemotherapy, immunotherapy, and targeted therapies.

10. Infectious Diseases: Infectious disease specialists deal with infections caused by bacteria, viruses, fungi, and parasites, including HIV, tuberculosis, and influenza.

11. Geriatrics: Geriatricians provide specialized care for older adults, addressing age-related health concerns and managing multiple medical conditions in the elderly population.

12. Hospital Medicine: Hospitalists focus on caring for patients during their hospital stay, coordinating with specialists and managing complex medical cases.

13. Critical Care Medicine: Critical care physicians manage patients in intensive care units (ICUs), providing specialized care for critically ill patients with life-threatening conditions.

14. Allergy and Immunology: Allergists and immunologists diagnose and treat allergic reactions, asthma, and immune system disorders.

15. Sports Medicine: Sports medicine

physicians manage injuries and medical conditions related to physical activity and sports participation.

16. Travel Medicine: Travel medicine specialists provide advice and vaccinations for individuals traveling to different regions, protecting against travel-related illnesses.

17. Occupational Medicine: Occupational medicine physicians focus on the health and safety of workers, addressing work-related injuries and illnesses.

18. Addiction Medicine: Addiction medicine specialists treat substance use disorders and provide support for individuals with addictions.

This list is by no means exhaustive, as internal medicine is a continuously evolving field that adapts to new medical advancements and patient needs. Internal medicine physicians, also known as internists, play a critical role in providing primary and specialized care for adult patients, helping to improve health outcomes and overall well-being.

The Importance of Interdisciplinary Collaboration in Healthcare

Interdisciplinary collaboration in healthcare is crucial for providing comprehensive, patient-centered, and effective care. It involves professionals from various healthcare disciplines working together as a team to address the complex needs of patients. Here are some key reasons why interdisciplinary collaboration is essential in healthcare:

1. Holistic Patient Care: Interdisciplinary teams take into account all aspects of a patient's health, including physical, mental, and social factors. This holistic approach leads to more comprehensive and personalized care.

2. Improved Patient Outcomes: Collaboration among healthcare professionals allows for better coordination of care, leading to improved patient outcomes and reduced medical errors.

3. Efficient Healthcare Delivery: Interdisciplinary teams streamline healthcare processes and avoid duplication of efforts, resulting in more efficient and cost-effective care.

4. Enhanced Communication: Collaborative teams promote effective communication among professionals, reducing misunderstandings and ensuring that everyone involved is on the same page regarding patient care.

5. Knowledge Sharing: Different disciplines bring unique expertise and perspectives to the table, promoting

knowledge sharing and continuous learning among team members.

6. Patient Education and Empowerment: Collaboration enables better patient education and empowerment, as patients receive information and guidance from multiple professionals who can address their diverse needs.

7. Continuity of Care: Collaborative care ensures smoother transitions between different healthcare settings and helps maintain continuity of care for patients.

8. Interprofessional Learning: Collaborative environments foster interprofessional learning, allowing healthcare professionals to understand and respect the roles and contributions of other disciplines.

9. Complex Cases and Comorbidities: In cases where patients have multiple chronic conditions or complex medical needs, interdisciplinary collaboration ensures that all aspects of their health are addressed.

10. Research and Innovation: Collaborative teams often engage in research and innovation, leading to advancements in medical treatments and care delivery.

11. Prevention and Health Promotion: Working together, healthcare professionals can better focus on preventive care and health promotion, which can lead to improved population health.

12. Ethical Decision Making: Interdisciplinary teams can navigate complex ethical issues more effectively, making decisions that prioritize the well-being of the patient.

In summary, interdisciplinary collaboration is essential for delivering high-quality healthcare. By combining the knowledge and skills of professionals from different disciplines, healthcare teams can provide more comprehensive, patient-centered, and efficient care, ultimately leading to better health outcomes for patients.

Final Thoughts and Call to Advancing Medical Expertise

As we conclude this journey through various medical specialties and healthcare disciplines, it is clear that the field of medicine is vast and continually evolving. The depth and breadth of medical knowledge and expertise required to provide effective patient care are immense. However, with advancements in technology, research, and interdisciplinary collaboration, healthcare professionals are better equipped than ever to meet the complex and diverse needs of patients.

It is essential for healthcare professionals to stay committed to lifelong learning and continuous professional development. As medical knowledge grows, new treatment modalities emerge, and best practices evolve, it is incumbent upon us to remain current and up-to-date. Embracing a growth mindset and seeking opportunities for learning and training will not only improve patient outcomes but also foster personal and professional fulfillment.

The call to advancing medical expertise extends to all healthcare professionals, from physicians, nurses, and therapists to medical assistants, technicians, and administrators. By working collaboratively and leveraging each other's strengths, we can create a more integrated and patient-centered healthcare system.

Moreover, we must recognize the significance of empathy, compassion, and cultural sensitivity in patient care. Treating patients as individuals, with respect and dignity, not only fosters better doctor-patient relationships but also plays a crucial role in healing and recovery.

In the face of the ever-changing landscape of healthcare, embracing innovation and embracing technology responsibly will be instrumental in improving healthcare access and quality. Telemedicine, artificial intelligence, data analytics, and other digital health solutions have the potential to revolutionize healthcare delivery and patient outcomes.

As healthcare professionals, our primary goal should always be to prioritize patient well-being and safety. This requires us to be advocates for evidence-based practices, patient rights, and ethical decision-making. Together, we can create a healthcare environment that ensures equitable access to high-quality care for all individuals.

Lastly, we should celebrate the diversity of healthcare professions and the contributions of each discipline in improving patient health and well-being. Recognizing and respecting the expertise and perspectives of our colleagues enhances interprofessional collaboration and fosters a more cohesive and integrated healthcare system.

In conclusion, let us remain committed to the pursuit of knowledge, the advancement of medical expertise, and the delivery of compassionate and patient-centered care. By working together, we can overcome challenges, seize opportunities, and continue to elevate the field of medicine to new heights. The impact we make as healthcare professionals reaches far beyond the clinic or hospital walls; it touches and transforms lives. Let us carry forward this knowledge and dedication as we strive for a healthier, more compassionate, and equitable world for all.

Glossary of Key Terms

Here's a glossary of key terms related to the field of medicine and healthcare:

1. Acute: Refers to a condition or illness that has a sudden onset and usually resolves within a short period.
2. Chronic: Describes a condition or illness that persists over a long duration, often for months or years.
3. Diagnosis: The identification of a disease or condition based on signs, symptoms, and medical tests.
4. Treatment: Medical interventions aimed at managing, curing, or alleviating symptoms of a disease or condition.
5. Prognosis: The expected outcome or course of a disease based on the current condition and treatment.
6. Symptom: A subjective indication of a disease or condition reported by the patient, such as pain or fatigue.
7. Sign: An objective indication of a disease or condition observed by a healthcare professional, such as a rash or fever.
8. Pathology: The study of diseases, their causes, and the effects on the body's organs and tissues.
9. Diagnosis: The identification of a disease or condition based on signs, symptoms, and medical tests.
10. Radiography: The use of X-rays to produce images of the internal structures of the body, commonly used for diagnosing bone fractures and dental problems.
11. Physical Therapy: A rehabilitation specialty

that uses physical techniques, exercises, and modalities to improve mobility and function.

12.   Occupational Therapy: A rehabilitation specialty that focuses on helping people with physical, mental, or cognitive disabilities regain independence and perform everyday tasks.

13.   Speech Therapy: A rehabilitation specialty that helps individuals with communication and swallowing disorders.

14.   Anesthesia: The administration of drugs to induce loss of sensation or consciousness during medical procedures.

15.   Surgery: Medical procedures that involve incisions or manipulation of body tissues to treat or diagnose a condition.

16.   Intensive Care Unit (ICU): A specialized medical unit that provides critical care and continuous monitoring for patients with severe illnesses or injuries.

17.   Telemedicine: The use of telecommunications technology to provide healthcare services remotely.

18.   Rehabilitation: The process of restoring individuals to their optimal physical, mental, and social functioning after an illness or injury.

19.   Preventive Medicine: Medical practices aimed at preventing diseases and promoting overall health and well-being.

20.   Infection Control: Measures taken to prevent the spread of infectious diseases within healthcare settings.

21.   Endocrinology: The study of hormones and their role in regulating various physiological processes in the body.

22.   Cardiology: The medical specialty that deals with the study and treatment of heart and

circulatory system disorders.

23.	Orthopedics: The branch of medicine dealing with the prevention and correction of injuries or disorders of the musculoskeletal system.

24.	Neurology: The medical specialty that deals with disorders of the nervous system, including the brain, spinal cord, and nerves.

25.	Hematology: The study of blood and blood-related disorders.

26.	Gastroenterology: The medical specialty that focuses on the digestive system and its disorders.

27.	Obstetrics & Gynecology (OB/GYN): The medical specialty dealing with women's reproductive health and childbirth.

28.	Geriatrics: The branch of medicine focused on the healthcare of elderly individuals.

29.	Pulmonology: The medical specialty dealing with the respiratory system and its disorders.

30.	Nephrology: The medical specialty dealing with the kidneys and their disorders.

This glossary includes some common terms, but the field of medicine is vast and continually evolving. Different medical specialties have their own specific terms and jargon. As healthcare professionals, staying updated with the latest terminologies and medical advancements is essential for effective communication and patient care.

List of Acronyms

Here is a list of commonly used acronyms in the medical and healthcare field:

1. CPR: Cardiopulmonary Resuscitation
2. MRI: Magnetic Resonance Imaging
3. CT: Computed Tomography
4. CBC: Complete Blood Count
5. HIV: Human Immunodeficiency Virus
6. AIDS: Acquired Immunodeficiency Syndrome
7. COVID-19: Coronavirus Disease 2019
8. ICU: Intensive Care Unit
9. ER: Emergency Room
10. ENT: Ear, Nose, and Throat
11. UTI: Urinary Tract Infection
12. CVA: Cerebrovascular Accident (Stroke)
13. COPD: Chronic Obstructive Pulmonary Disease
14. DM: Diabetes Mellitus
15. CHF: Congestive Heart Failure
16. AMI: Acute Myocardial Infarction (Heart Attack)
17. BP: Blood Pressure
18. BMI: Body Mass Index
19. GERD: Gastroesophageal Reflux Disease
20. C-section: Cesarean Section
21. TIA: Transient Ischemic Attack (Mini-Stroke)
22. CABG: Coronary Artery Bypass Graft
23. PTCA: Percutaneous Transluminal

Coronary Angioplasty
24.   RA: Rheumatoid Arthritis
25.   CVA: Cerebrovascular Accident (Stroke)
26.   GI: Gastrointestinal
27.   ENT: Ear, Nose, and Throat
28.   MS: Multiple Sclerosis
29.   EBV: Epstein-Barr Virus
30.   CBC: Complete Blood Count
31.   MRI: Magnetic Resonance Imaging
32.   WBC: White Blood Cell
33.   HbA1c: Glycated Hemoglobin (Blood Sugar Level)
34.   LDL: Low-Density Lipoprotein
35.   HDL: High-Density Lipoprotein
36.   PSA: Prostate-Specific Antigen
37.   NSAIDs: Nonsteroidal Anti-Inflammatory Drugs
38.   NPO: Nothing by Mouth (Nil Per Os)
39.   PO: By Mouth (Per Os)
40.   IV: Intravenous
41.   IM: Intramuscular
42.   BP: Blood Pressure
43.   HR: Heart Rate
44.   RR: Respiratory Rate
45.   CNS: Central Nervous System
46.   PPE: Personal Protective Equipment
47.   HIPAA: Health Insurance Portability and Accountability Act
48.   EMR: Electronic Medical Record
49.   EHR: Electronic Health Record
50.   HIP: History, Inspection, Palpation (Medical Examination)

Please note that this list includes some of the most common acronyms, but there are many more used in the medical field. As healthcare professionals, it is important to be familiar with these acronyms to facilitate effective communication in the workplace.

References and Recommended Readings

Some reputable sources for medical and healthcare information:

1. Centers for Disease Control and Prevention (CDC) - cdc.gov
2. World Health Organization (WHO) - who.int
3. National Institutes of Health (NIH) - nih.gov
4. Mayo Clinic - mayoclinic.org
5. WebMD - webmd.com
6. American Medical Association (AMA) - ama-assn.org
7. National Health Service (NHS) - nhs.uk (for UK healthcare information)
8. Medscape - medscape.com

For specific medical topics, it's always best to consult peer-reviewed medical journals, textbooks, and trusted medical professionals.

Keep in mind that medical information should be obtained from reliable sources, and it's important to verify information with healthcare professionals, especially for personalized medical advice and treatment.